AIDS

images of the epidemic

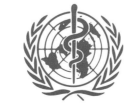

World Health Organization

Geneva

1994

WHO Library Cataloguing in Publication Data

AIDS : images of the epidemic.

1.Acquired immunodeficiency syndrome - epidemiology
2.Acquired immunodeficiency syndrome - statistics
3.HIV infections

ISBN 92 4 156163 7   (NLM Classification: WD 308)

Contents

Preface

Ten years ago, the acronym "AIDS" was barely known. By 1993, over 2.5 million people worldwide had developed the fatal condition denoted by those four letters. And the global epidemic continues to expand. Every day, the virus that causes AIDS infects well over 5000 people — most of them young or middle-aged adults on whom families, communities and economies depend. By the end of this decade, a cumulative total of 40 million people may have been infected — more than all those killed in the Second World War.

By setting out some of the facts, figures and faces of the epidemic this book aims to provide not an exhaustive account but rather snapshots of AIDS today, drawing on first-hand experiences, mainly in Ethiopia, Thailand, the United Republic of Tanzania and the United Kingdom. Many of the images are grim, but there *are* grounds for hope.

After a brief account of what is currently known about the syndrome called AIDS, the dynamics of the epidemic are described, region by region, in order to show where AIDS is and where it is heading. This section, printed on coloured paper, is essentially for reference, and readers who are less interested in the statistics than in the discussion may wish to pass over it.

Why is it that thousands of people are still becoming infected every day, despite prevention campaigns undertaken by national AIDS programmes worldwide? There are many answers to this question, for AIDS is mainly a sexually transmitted disease and the spread of the virus is fuelled by taboos, complacency, ignorance, and a host of other factors. In this book, we analyse just a few of them: discrimination and denial, poverty, and inequality between the sexes.

But many people are meeting the challenge of AIDS with courage, resourcefulness and often remarkable success, and their stories — again, mostly from the four countries mentioned earlier — are told in the last part of the book. Even though there is neither vaccine nor cure, experience shows that the millions of uninfected men, women and children in the world *can* be protected from the virus and the millions with HIV infection or AIDS given compassionate, dignified care.

Note: *Any attempt to describe AIDS — an epidemic as volatile as the human response to it — is inevitably fraught with difficulty. Where this book's descriptions are already out of date, we apologize: our intention in quoting individuals and citing examples within selected countries was simply to illustrate important points.*

Acknowledgements

WHO wishes to thank Sue Armstrong, a science writer specializing in health issues, for her invaluable contribution to this book. As a journalist, she travelled in Ethiopia, Thailand, the United Republic of Tanzania and the United Kingdom to interview the people whose stories bring this picture of the epidemic to life.

The Organization is grateful to many people for the help, kindness and cooperation they extended to Sue Armstrong and to the photographers — Gérard Diez and Louise Gubb — who travelled with her. In particular, we would like to mention Almaz G./Kidane, Fikerte Belete and Hawulte Begoayehu (Ethiopia), Nuntawun Yuntadilok (Thailand), and Protase Karani, Ismail Mwishashi and Odelia Rwenyagira (United Republic of Tanzania).

Lastly, WHO wishes to acknowledge the generous financial contribution of the Sasakawa Memorial Health Foundation which made possible the publication of this book.

PART I
What is AIDS?

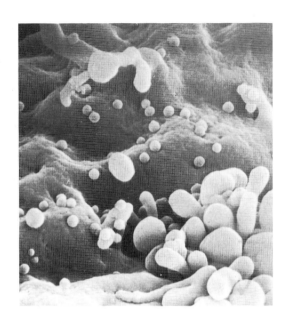

CHAPTER 1

The early days

"In June of 1981 we saw a young gay man with the most devastating immune deficiency we had ever seen. We said, 'We don't know what this is, but we hope we don't ever see another case like it again'." — *Dr Samuel Broder, USA (1)*

On the trail of a new disease

In 1979, two young men from New York City visited their doctors with symptoms of a rare tumour, Kaposi sarcoma. Similar diagnoses had been made in young men in other US cities, and cases of another rare disease — *Pneumocystis carinii* pneumonia — had been making their appearance independently in various parts of the country. It took their puzzled doctors a while to realize that these scattered mysteries were part of a trend.

It then fell to epidemiologists — or "medical detectives" — to piece together the picture. What was causing these rare conditions in previously healthy young men? Two facts linked the cases: all the patients were homosexual, and their diseases indicated a drastically weakened immune system.

Epidemiologists ask themselves what differentiates people who fall ill from those who remain well. What most appeared to distinguish early AIDS patients was their homosexuality, so scientists began looking for clues in their lifestyles. (For a short time in the USA, the syndrome was called gay-related immune deficiency, or GRID.) The use of inhalant "poppers" — stimulant drugs based on amyl nitrite — was widespread in sections of the gay community in the United States of America at the time, and scientists wondered whether these could have caused the men's immune systems to collapse. The observation that AIDS was more common among men who had many sex partners, sexually transmitted diseases (STDs) and intestinal infections, led to a second theory: the men might be overburdening their immune systems to the point of collapse. Unexpected appearances of *Pneumocystis carinii* pneumonia and Kaposi sarcoma among injecting drug users did nothing to undermine this hypothesis, as initially it was argued that hepatitis B and other infections caused by needle-sharing might similarly overload the immune system.

Soon, however, the ailments characteristic of the new syndrome began to show up among men with haemophilia — who suffer through heredity from the absence of factor VIII, an essential clotting factor in the blood — and among men, women and children who had received blood transfusions. Haemophilia is treated with factor VIII extracted from the pooled blood of thousands of donors. So the evidence now pointed to an infectious agent carried in blood.

In other parts of the world, too, doctors were beginning to witness similarly baffling outbreaks of disease. "I well remember a medical meeting we had in 1981," says Dr Katende Kashaija, Medical Officer for Kagera Region in the United Republic of Tanzania. "The guest of honour was the regional commissioner and he alerted us to the fact that there was a strange disease around which the people were calling 'hella's disease'. *Hella* is a Swahili word meaning 'money' and they called it that because they noticed it was rich traders and fishermen who were coming down with it.

"We physicians thought this was a funny thing: we'd never read anything about a 'disease of money' in our textbooks. So we asked the District Medical Officer to investigate in the places where it was reported — along the border between Tanzania and Uganda. He came back eventually with a report that the problem was *lymphogranuloma venereum*, a sexually transmitted disease which causes swelling in the groin. But as months went by we saw that the disease was spreading, and that it was appearing with more and more complicated manifestations. It was about that time that we started to read reports from the USA about a similar phenomenon."

As realization dawned that patients with clusters of disease similar to those seen in the USA were appearing in Africa, Australia and Europe, doctors began to recall having seen syndromes of this kind in the late 1970s. A few such cases were described from even earlier periods — as far back as 1959.

But what was the causal infectious agent?

The world was fortunate indeed that by the time this became a burning question, a great deal had been learnt about the retroviruses — a large family of viruses to which the virus that causes AIDS belongs. In the USA, Professor Howard Temin and Professor David Baltimore laid the first cornerstone for the discovery of the human immunodeficiency virus (HIV) with their detection of the crucial enzyme reverse transcriptase, for which they were later honoured with the Nobel Prize. Dr Robert Gallo, in identifying the retrovirus known as HTLV-1, then developed many of the techniques that would make HIV's discovery possible.

The first photographs of HIV were taken with an electron microscope in February 1983, at the Pasteur Institute in Paris, where a French research team led by Professor Luc Montagnier had isolated the virus in tissue taken from a young homosexual man with chronically swollen lymph glands. Several months later, Montagnier and his colleagues Dr Françoise Barré-Sinoussi and Dr Jean-Claude Chermann published a description of HIV. They believed, rightly, that they had found the causal agent of AIDS.

Gearing up to fight AIDS

As the 1980s wore on, and AIDS appeared in men, women and children throughout the world, public health experts realized that they were dealing with a lethal syndrome that was far more widespread and fast-moving than first believed.

As awareness grew of the threat posed by AIDS, so did the urgent need for a global response to bolster the grass-roots campaigns initiated by communities hard hit by the epidemic. The first international meeting on AIDS was convened by WHO in late 1983; it was to be followed by many more in subsequent years. Immediately after the First In-

Extraordinary energies have emerged at local and national levels in response to AIDS and a constellation of truly remarkable and exceptionally dedicated people, throughout the world, have risen to the scientific, public health, political and human challenges of AIDS." — Dr Jonathan M. Mann, Director, WHO Special Programme on AIDS (2)

ternational Conference on AIDS, held in 1985 in Atlanta, USA, a group of scientists and health professionals met under the auspices of WHO to make recommendations on how to prevent the further spread of AIDS. Later that year, WHO organized the first meeting on AIDS in Africa, held in Bangui, Central African Republic, to establish clinical criteria for the reporting of cases. No laboratory test for HIV infection or AIDS had yet been developed, but it was urgent to know more about the scope and spread of the epidemic. At the same time, WHO was drafting a global strategy for the prevention and control of AIDS, setting forth the main action needed and the principles that should govern the international response. This strategy was endorsed unanimously by the World Health Assembly in May 1987 and formally adopted in September by the United Nations General Assembly.

WHO's Special Programme on AIDS, later called the Global Programme on AIDS (GPA), had already begun to work with individual countries, helping them with short-term measures for responding to the crisis and then with support for a national AIDS programme capable of taking on long-term prevention, control and care. Today, national AIDS programmes have been established in virtually every country of the world — most of them guided by the global AIDS strategy (which was updated in 1992) and with advice from WHO.

CHAPTER 2

HIV infection and AIDS

"I have a face in my mind for every AIDS-related condition I can describe to you, and sometimes several faces, every one the face of a friend either living or dead. I can see little quick relief from the cycle of sickness and death that for over a decade now has drained my community and rendered our culture incalculably poorer." — *Jim Eigo, USA (3)*

HIV — a slow-acting virus

Most viruses produce their major impact in a matter of days or weeks. The influenza virus, for example, causes flu within 1–5 days; hepatitis A takes about 4 weeks to develop after infection.

HIV is different. Except for a generally mild illness (fever, sore throat and rash) that about 70% of people experience a few weeks after initial infection with the virus, most HIV-infected people have no symptoms for the first five or so years. They look healthy and feel well — although right from the start they can transmit the virus to others. Once infected, people are infected for life. Scientists have not as yet found a way of curing them, or making them uninfectious to others. Current evidence suggests that, in the absence of other causes of death, almost all HIV-infected people will ultimately die of AIDS.

Soon after a person is infected with HIV, the immune system produces antibodies in an attempt to neutralize the virus. As antibodies to HIV are far easier to detect than the virus itself, their presence or absence in the bloodstream is the basis for the most widely used test of HIV infection. A person whose blood contains HIV antibodies is said to be HIV-positive, or seropositive, meaning that he or she is infected with HIV.

HIV antibodies usually take between two weeks and three months to appear in the bloodstream, though they have been known to take longer. The period before antibodies are produced is the "window period" during which — although the person is particularly infectious because of the high concentration of virus in the blood — he or she will test negative on the standard antibody blood tests.

Though the body's immune system reacts to the invasion of HIV by producing anti-bodies, these do not inactivate the virus in the usual way. In fact, the virus attacks key cells in the immune system and causes a gradual breakdown in the body's defences against other infections (see panel, p. 6).

HIV-2

In the early 1980s, a number of cases with all the characteristics of AIDS — but which turned out not to be caused by HIV — appeared in people from parts of west Africa. One of the patients was a Portuguese man who had lived all his life on the Cape Verde islands, 800 km off the coast of Senegal. In 1982 he developed symptoms of AIDS for which he eventually sought treatment in Paris. In 1985 scientists managed to isolate the virus that was causing the man's illness. Viewed with an electron microscope it had an appearance uncharacteristic of HIV, but further investigation revealed that it was a variant of the first human immunodeficiency virus. It was later named HIV-2.

HIV-2 appears to be slightly different in genetic make-up from what, ever since, has been known as HIV-1. It attacks the immune system in the same way, and makes infected people vulnerable to the same opportunistic infections, though research has suggested that people infected with HIV-2 progress more slowly towards AIDS. So far, most AIDS cases resulting from HIV-2 have been in people living in west Africa, but cases have also been found on other continents.

The illnesses called AIDS

AIDS stands for acquired immunodeficiency syndrome. It is not a single disease; it is the end stage of infection with HIV, charac-

HIV and the immune system

The body cells that are the main targets of HIV are T-helper lymphocytes and the scavenger cells known as monocytes, which turn into macrophages when they leave the bloodstream to enter a body organ. In a healthy immune system, the monocytes/macrophages defend the body by seeking out and eliminating foreign particles and dead or infected cells. The body also defends itself by manufacturing special proteins called antibodies to render foreign bodies (known collectively as antigens) harmless. HIV infection interferes with both these processes, gradually weakening the immune system.

The cells that produce antibodies are a type of lymphocyte (white blood cell) known as B cells. These cells manufacture antibodies specific to the antigen they seek to destroy, and some retain a memory of the antigen they have encountered, which enables the immune system to react swiftly if the antigen should reappear even years later.

Other important lymphocytes in the immune system are the T cells, which circulate in the bloodstream and concentrate at sites of invasion by a foreign body. Besides serving as specialized killers and helping B cells to make antibodies, the T cells coordinate the immune system's response to an antigen and switch the system off when danger is past. Some T cells, too, retain a memory of antigens they have encountered.

The T cell that regulates and coordinates the other cells is called a T-helper cell. It is the main target of HIV. The virus breaks into the cell and throws the whole immune system into chaos by sidelining all the other cells dependent on the T-helper cell. (The T-helper cell — whose full name is the CD4+ T lymphocyte — is also commonly known as a CD4+ cell.) HIV further outwits the immune system by changing constantly and becoming unrecognizable to antibodies produced against it.

Once inside the CD4+ cell, HIV uses the host cell's machinery to reproduce rapidly and massively. The new viruses form buds on the surface of the host cell before bursting into the bloodstream to invade other cells. A very low number of CD4+ cells in the blood indicates an impaired immune system and means a person is unable to fight off diseases or infections that would normally pose little threat.

HIV is also attracted to monocytes/macrophages but it does not destroy them in the same way as it does the CD4+ cells. Instead, it hides in them and is carried to the brain, lungs and other parts of the body, particularly the lymph nodes.

terized by a cluster — or "syndrome" — of life-threatening illnesses. While people with AIDS can be helped with medicines, there is as yet no cure, and most people die within one to three years after diagnosis.

In some people the period between infection with HIV and the development of AIDS may be a few years; in others it is 10 years or more. Intensive research is being conducted to find out the reasons for these variations. Scientists believe they could be due to differences in the aggressivity (virulence) of different HIV strains, or in individuals' genetic make-up or immune response; or to the presence of other diseases that might accelerate the infectious process. Disease progression is especially swift in infants and young children: around four out of five become seriously ill or die before their fifth birthday.

Most HIV-infected people suffer intermittent bouts of illness that increase in severity as their immune systems collapse. Different disease-causing microorganisms break through the immune system at different stages. Doctors can tell approximately the state of the immune system from the symptoms presented by their HIV-infected patients. The number of CD4+ cells in the bloodstream can also give some indication of immune status.

> Humans live in relative harmony with a range of viruses, bacteria, parasites and fungi that do not cause disease in healthy people with intact immune defences. But these organisms can take advantage of someone with a weakened immune system, such as an individual infected with HIV. The infections they cause are thus known as *opportunistic infections.*

The course of HIV infection can be divided into several stages, only the last of which is defined as AIDS. In the earliest stage, an HIV-infected person may be asymptomatic except for swollen lymph nodes in the neck, armpits and groin which do not make the person feel ill but may prompt a visit to the doctor.

As the infection progresses, the individual may suffer a range of conditions including intense fatigue, persistent cough and fever, profuse sweating at night, diarrhoea and dramatic loss of weight, skin rashes, mouth ulcers and oral thrush (a fungal infection of the mouth), herpes infections including shingles, and a normally rare condition known as oral hairy leukoplakia which appears as patches of white warts on the side of the tongue and inside the cheek.

People with a healthy immune system usually have more than 950 CD4 + cells in each microlitre of blood, although a few people never have more than 500 and remain healthy.

The number of CD4 + cells usually falls over the course of HIV infection. People with AIDS usually have a CD4 + count of below 200. (The USA makes a CD4 + count of below 200 in an HIV-infected person a *definition* of AIDS.)

A number of opportunistic diseases commonly occur at this last stage of HIV infection known as AIDS. Tuberculosis (see panel below) and Kaposi sarcoma, a tumour that manifests itself as purple patches on the skin and internally, are usually seen relatively early, when the

Tuberculosis: new life in an old enemy

An alarming factor in the AIDS epidemic is the increasingly close link between HIV infection and tuberculosis (TB). TB, which flourishes in conditions of poverty and overcrowding, is endemic in much of the developing world and in poor urban ghettos of some developed countries.

In countries where TB is endemic, many people are infected in childhood. A healthy immune system usually keeps the infection in check, and people may remain infected for life with dormant and uninfectious TB. (Such people are called TB carriers.) But if the immune system breaks down — as it does among people with HIV infection — the TB can become active. This means the people develop the disease and at the same time become contagious to others with whom they come into close contact. Studies in Rwanda, the USA, Zaire and Zambia found that HIV-positive individuals were 30 – 50 times more likely to develop active TB than HIV-negative people.

As a consequence, AIDS is reviving an old problem in developed countries, e.g. in the USA, where a long-standing annual decline in TB cases ended abruptly in 1985. In developing countries, where up to 80% of adults in the poorest, most overcrowded cities are TB carriers, AIDS is exacerbating an existing problem. In some African countries, cases of TB have doubled or even tripled since 1985. According to WHO figures, up to half of all people in Africa newly diagnosed as having pulmonary TB are also HIV-positive. So the communities in which TB carriers live — developing countries and the poor inner cities of the developed world — face parallel epidemics of AIDS and TB once HIV is introduced.

The problem is compounded by the fact that in these same communities many TB patients do not complete the full course of treatment, thus permitting the emergence of TB bacilli that are resistant to the commonly used anti-tuberculosis drugs. Patients who have clinical disease caused by drug-resistant bacilli are as contagious as those with drug-sensitive TB, almost untreatable, and likely to increase in number. Several outbreaks of drug-resistant tuberculosis have already been reported.

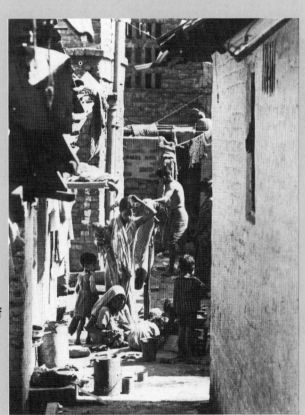

Up to 80% of adults in the poorest and most overcrowded cities of the world carry tuberculosis — an infection which often becomes activated and contagious in a person whose immune system is weakened by HIV. Today, many countries face parallel epidemics of TB and AIDS.

CD4 + count is still above 100. Serious fungal infections (such as *Candida* oesophagitis, *Cryptococcus* meningitis, and penicillosis) and parasitic infections (e.g. *Pneumocystis carinii* pneumonia or *Toxoplasma gondii* encephalitis) tend to occur when the CD4 + count has dropped to around 100. People whose counts are below 50 have the late opportunistic infections such as cytomegaloviral retinitis.

Many people with AIDS are affected by a wasting syndrome that is known, especially in Africa, as "slim disease". It involves chronic diarrhoea and severe weight loss. Another condition seen worldwide is AIDS encephalopathy or AIDS dementia, which is caused by HIV crossing the so-called "blood-brain barrier", which normally keeps foreign agents from reaching the brain. In its late stages, AIDS encephalopathy resembles senile dementia or Alzheimer disease. AIDS dementia appears to result not from opportunistic infection but from the action of the virus itself.

CHAPTER 3

HIV transmission: matters of fact

Fortunately for the human race, HIV does not spread through water, food or air. If it did, our species might be threatened with extinction.

HIV spreads primarily through sexual intercourse, which makes HIV infection basically a sexually transmitted disease (STD). Like some other STDs, HIV can also be transmitted through infected blood, blood products, and transplanted organs and tissues (including sperm), and from a mother to her fetus or baby.

Sexual transmission

"Epidemics are not accidents", said Dr Nathan Clumek of St Pierre Hospital, Brussels, who was one of the first physicians to describe AIDS in heterosexuals (4). "A new pathogen will enter a community only when the conditions are ripe for it."

In a world where an estimated 250 million people a year acquire an STD, including gonorrhoea, syphilis, chancroid, genital warts (papilloma) and genital herpes, it will readily be appreciated that there is ample opportunity for the spread of HIV. In many countries, HIV infection has appeared first among people with the most sex partners, although it is only a matter of time before the virus finds its way outside these circles. Sexual transmission accounts for approximately 75% of all HIV infections worldwide.

Global HIV infections in 1993

Mode of transmission

Sexual intercourse	70–80%
Mother to child	5–10%
Needle-sharing by drug users	5–10%
Blood transfusion	3–5%
Accidental needle-sticks to health care workers	less than 0.01%

Every single act of unprotected intercourse (i.e. intercourse without a condom) with an HIV-infected person exposes the uninfected partner to the risk of infection. The size of the risk is affected by a number of factors, including the presence of other STDs, the sex and age of the uninfected partner, the type of sexual act, the stage of illness of the infected partner, and the virulence of the HIV strain involved.

A European study of 563 heterosexual couples in which only one partner was infected at the start suggested that transmission from male to female was about twice as likely as from female to male (5). Generally, women are more vulnerable to HIV infection because a larger surface (the vagina and cervix) is exposed. Moreover, semen contains a far higher concentration of HIV than do vaginal and cervical fluids.

Anal intercourse, whether between man and woman or between men, carries a higher risk of transmission than vaginal intercourse because it is more likely to injure the tissues of the receptive partner. Again, as for vaginal sex, the receptive partner is at greater risk than the insertive partner.

Since both semen and vaginal fluid contain HIV, there is a theoretical risk of transmission through oral sex — both cunnilingus and fellatio. The actual risk is difficult to measure scientifically: few people engage in oral sex to the exclusion of all other practices, and if they become infected the route of transmission is unclear. Oral sex does, however, appear to pose far less of a risk of HIV transmission than vaginal or anal intercourse. This helps explain the rarity of HIV transmission through sex between women.

For all forms of sex, the risk of transmission is greater where there are abrasions of the skin or mucous membrane. For oral and vaginal sex, the risk is greater when the woman is menstruating.

Age appears to be a factor in the susceptibility of women, making them more vulnerable to HIV infection in their teens and again when over the age of 45. In adolescent women the immature cervix is thought to be a less efficient barrier to HIV than the mature

Reducing HIV transmission through blood and blood products

Today, WHO estimates that the risk in industrialized countries of acquiring HIV infection from the transfusion of donated blood or blood products is around 1 in 100 000, or even less, for each unit of blood transfused. People with haemophilia should no longer be at risk: a process of heat-treating factor VIII has been developed that kills HIV and other viruses. (Unfortunately, whole blood cannot be heat-treated to kill HIV.) A synthetic factor VIII is also now on the market.

In some parts of the developing world, however, it has proved more difficult to ensure blood safety. The main problems are inadequate organization of blood transfusion services, a lack of trained staff, and insufficient funds.

Full protection of the blood supply means building in safety measures at every stage and not relying wholly on the HIV antibody test, which cannot detect infection in blood during the "window period" between infection and the appearance of antibodies. The initial supply of blood needs to be as infection-free as possible. Blood transfusion services should therefore discourage donations from people who might be infected (although this is difficult wherever donors are paid or otherwise rewarded for giving blood) and encourage voluntary unpaid donations from those at low risk of infection. In parallel, doctors and the prescribers of blood need to be educated not to give blood unnecessarily but to reserve it for life-threatening situations. In many instances, blood substitutes — salt solutions and colloids — can be given instead.

Estimated percentage of blood screened for HIV antibody, by country, 1992

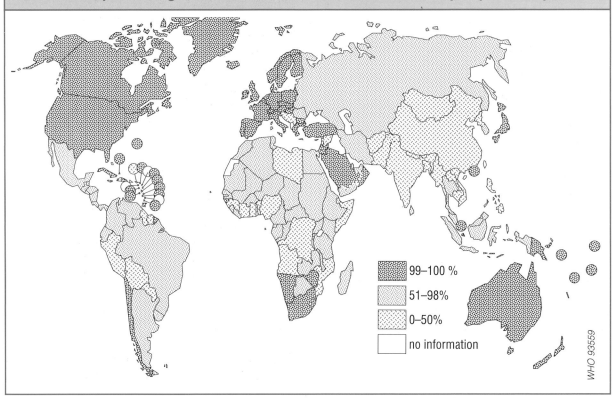

99–100 %

51–98%

0–50%

no information

WHO 93559

genital tract of older women. And the thinning and drying of the vaginal mucosa at the menopause is believed to lessen the barrier effect for women who have reached this stage in life. The production of mucus in the genital tract of adolescent girls and postmenopausal women is not as prolific as in women between these life stages, and this may also enhance their susceptibility to HIV infection.

As for HIV-infected people, they are more infectious to others in the very early stages — before antibody production (i.e. during the "window period") — and when infection is well advanced, because levels of virus in the blood are higher then than at other times.

An important biological factor affecting the probability of HIV transmission is the presence of another sexually transmitted disease.

An STD in either the HIV-negative or the HIV-positive partner facilitates the transmission of HIV:

- If an STD, such as syphilis, chancroid or herpes, causes ulceration in the genital or perineal area of the uninfected partner, it becomes far easier for HIV to pass into his or her tissues. Studies suggest that the risk increases many-fold.
- For a person with a non-ulcerative STD such as gonorrhoea or chlamydial infection, there is also an increased risk.
- An STD causes inflammation: T cells and monocytes/macrophages, sent to check the infection, concentrate in the genital area. In a person already infected with HIV, some of these key cells of the immune system will be carrying the virus — which magnifies the risk of transmission to the uninfected partner.

Ways of reducing HIV spread through sex

- abstinence from sex
- mutual fidelity (between uninfected partners)
- forms of sex not involving penetration
- condom use for all forms of penetrative sex

It cannot be overemphasized that even small risks add up to danger when they occur again and again. "It's like crossing a busy highway on foot", says Dr Jim Chin, former chief of epidemiological surveillance for GPA. "The risk is small with each crossing, so you may take the chance and get away with it 10 times, maybe even 100 times. If you keep on crossing the highway, you'll get run over."

Ways of reducing HIV spread through drug use

- abstinence from drug use
- switch from injection to safer forms of drug use (oral, inhaled)
- avoidance of needle-sharing with others
- use of sterile injection equipment for each dose
- cleaning of injection equipment with bleach

products, such as untreated factor VIII administered to people with haemophilia.

Intact skin is an effective barrier against the virus. When it is pierced by needles, tattooing equipment or other invasive instruments that have been contaminated with blood containing HIV, infection can take place if the "dose" of virus is large enough. A small possibility exists that bloodborne virus might enter the body through a mucous membrane — by blood spurting into the eye during surgery, for example. There is a tiny theoretical risk of infection from a contaminated razor blade, but transmission via this route has not been documented.

Since the likelihood of HIV transmission through blood depends on the "dose" of virus injected, the risk of getting infected through a contaminated needle, syringe or any other skin-piercing instrument is very much lower than with transfusion. Nevertheless, among drug users who inject heroin, cocaine or other substances, this route of transmission is significant because exposure is repeated so often — in some cases, several times a day. As a result, needle-sharing by drug users is a major cause of AIDS in many countries, both developed and developing, and in some it is the predominant cause.

Blood

Contaminated blood is highly infective when introduced in large quantities directly into the bloodstream. The risk of contracting HIV infection from a transfusion of a unit of infected blood is estimated to be over 95%. HIV is also readily transmitted through infected blood

Mother-to-child transmission

HIV may pass from an infected woman to her fetus, or to her infant during delivery or breast-feeding (see panel). This is known as mother-to-child transmission, and around one-third of the children of HIV-infected mothers worldwide are infected through this route.

Breast is still best

Some mother-to-child infections occur through breast-feeding. So what does this mean for an infected woman soon to give birth? Should she, or should she not, breast-feed her baby? "A mother who knows she is infected has to weigh the risks of transmitting HIV to her baby through breast-feeding against the risks to the child of not breast-feeding," says Dr Susan Holck, chief of policy coordination for GPA. "In many settings babies have a very high chance of dying from diarrhoea or other infectious diseases if they are not breast-fed.

"For breast-milk substitutes to be even considered, an HIV-infected mother must be able to afford regular supplies of infant formula. She needs to be able to read and understand the mixing instructions. And she must have easy access to clean water."

In the light of all the evidence, WHO and UNICEF stress that breast-feeding remains the safest way to protect the health and lives of babies, including the vast majority of those born to HIV-positive mothers, and that the practice should be promoted, protected and supported in all countries, irrespective of their HIV prevalence.

Studies suggest that the risk of transmission from mother to infant is higher if the mother is newly infected, or if she has already developed AIDS, than if she has an established HIV infection without symptoms. Worldwide, 5–10% of all HIV infections in 1993 are thought to have been acquired through this route. Because infants and children progress so rapidly to AIDS, however, they already account for about 20% of AIDS cases to date.

Groundless fears

Ignorance about how HIV is transmitted — together with the fatal nature of AIDS and its association with taboo or condemned behaviour — has produced a cruel mixture of prejudice and discrimination. The epidemic abounds with stories not only of sick, wasted people and motherless children, but also of infected people finding their belongings on the street and their homes locked against them; of workers fired, children barred from school, and many lesser insults and indignities. So establishing how the virus is not transmitted is as important as establishing how it is.

In the laboratory, scientists have managed to isolate HIV in tears, sweat, urine and saliva, but only blood, semen, vaginal fluid and breast-milk have high enough concentrations of HIV to be infective. Furthermore, HIV must penetrate the skin or come into direct contact with a mucous membrane for infection to take place. So doorknobs, toilet seats, crockery, swimming pools and drinking fountains *cannot* transmit HIV. There is *no danger* in riding on a bus, sharing a meal or holding hands with people with AIDS, or even in hugging or cuddling.

Studies in many countries show that HIV does not spread through casual, everyday contact. For example, scientists in the USA studied 206 offspring, siblings, parents and friends sharing the home of someone who had AIDS (6). Most lived in overcrowded conditions especially conducive to the spread of infection. Yet even after close contact over an average of 23 months, not a single person tested had become infected with HIV, even though interactions included the sharing of items and facilities likely to be soiled with blood. There were thousands of days on which someone drank out of the same glass as the infected person, and thousands of occasions on which household members hugged, kissed, and shared baths and even beds (without sexual intercourse), without themselves becoming infected.

I remember the first time someone died at the house we started for people with AIDS two years ago. Ian belonged to a church which embalms the bodies of members who die. But when he died, his church refused to perform those rites. They just came along with a steel coffin inside a wooden one. At that stage no nurses would even come into the house, so we as sick people had to nurse each other. We had nursed Ian during his dying and now we had to lay his body in the coffin, too, and screw the lid down tight and give it to the undertakers all sealed. These guys stood outside, they wouldn't even come into the house.

"I think a lot of the prejudice and rejection is based on fear of the unknown."
— *Pietro Battiston (7)*

There were initially concerns that blood-sucking insects might transmit HIV in much the same way that they pass on malaria, dengue and yellow fever. But these fears have now been laid to rest. Epidemiological observation and laboratory work furnish clear evidence that *insects do not transmit HIV*.

For example, if mosquitos were vehicles for HIV transmission we would expect to find infection spread evenly throughout the population, with all age groups being equally affected. The epidemiological pattern of HIV infection is completely different. Cases are rare in people who are generally sexually inactive — youngsters under 15 years old (except for infants infected through their mothers) and very old people. And HIV infection rates tend to be lower in rural areas than in urban areas, though in many countries mosquitos are more plentiful in the countryside.

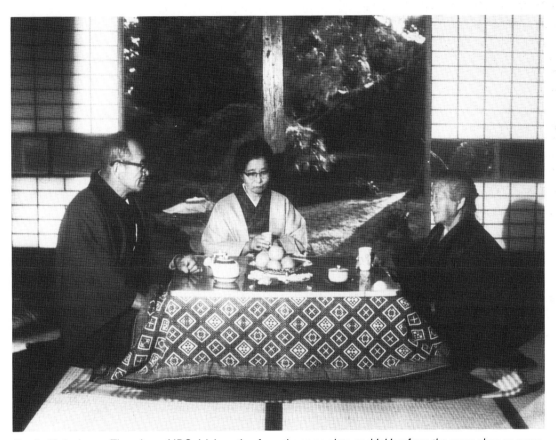

Family life in Japan. There is no AIDS risk in eating from the same plate or drinking from the same glass as someone infected with HIV. The virus simply does not spread that way.

PART II

AIDS: a global epidemic

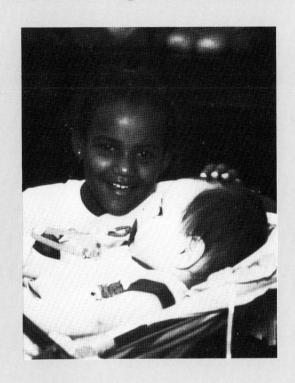

CHAPTER 4

What is known?

"HIV is dangerous because its workings remain invisible for so long. There is no ulceration, no serious symptom linked with initial infection. On average, worldwide, it takes 10 years to progress from initial infection to AIDS. The long time period between infection and illness is precious to each infected individual, but paradoxically it is a calamity when it comes to mass awareness." — Dr Hiroshi Nakajima, Director-General, WHO (8)

By late 1993, close to 850 000 cases of AIDS had been reported to WHO from over 180 countries and territories. For several reasons, however, this is thought to represent only a small proportion of the true world total. Many countries were slow to admit they had an AIDS problem and to set up systematic surveillance and reporting. Moreover, where expertise and blood testing facilities are lacking, it may be difficult to differentiate AIDS from other common diseases. And in remote parts of the developing world, many people fall ill and die without ever coming into contact with modern health services.

"Getting transport to bring a very sick person to hospital is often just too expensive for a family," says Mr A. Byashara, Regional AIDS Coordinator in Kagera, United Republic of Tanzania, an area with one of the world's highest AIDS prevalences. *"Besides, most people now know the symptoms of AIDS; many people don't even try to reach hospital if they believe they've got it because they think it's untreatable."*

Taking all these factors into account, WHO estimates that by early 1994 more than 3 million cases of AIDS had actually occurred, including over 500 000 in infants born to HIV-infected women.

But the number of AIDS cases gives a foretaste rather than a true reflection of the health crisis facing the world, for AIDS is the *late* stage of infection with a virus that takes many years — often more than a decade — to cause illness. The real measure of the scope of the epidemic is the number of people infected with HIV. Extrapolating from the data that are available, WHO estimates that about 1 million

children and more than 14 million young people and adults worldwide had been infected with HIV by early 1994, of whom about 12 million were still alive. By the turn of the century, if WHO's conservative forecasts prove correct, the cumulative total of HIV infections may reach 30–40 million and the number of AIDS cases more than 10 million.

HIV/AIDS does not affect populations uniformly, either at the global level or within any one country, and the epidemic is in reality the sum of many local epidemics. Each has its own distinctive characteristics shaped by local social, economic, cultural and similar factors. What, then, does the epidemic look like in different parts of the world?

The snapshots offered in the following chapters have been pieced together from the growing body of research data.[1] But it must be stressed that the information available is incomplete and sometimes hard to interpret. Because infected people often have no symptoms for many years, the traditional public health method of "case reporting" does not work for HIV infection. The best way to keep HIV spread under surveillance is to carry out periodic "unlinked" testing in selected population groups, i.e. HIV testing in which only the general characteristics of the people tested are recorded, not their names or any other identifying data, so as to preserve anonymity.

The most convenient approach to surveillance is to locate it in the health care system and test people who come in for care. Given that three-quarters of all HIV infections are sexually transmitted, some groups — such as people attending STD clinics — are likely to become infected earlier than others, and this is why they are often chosen as "sentinel" groups for surveillance. Another group that is useful

---

[1] A list of references and suggestions for further reading are available from the Global Programme on AIDS, World Health Organization, 1211 Geneva 27, Switzerland.

AIDS and sex work: what the statistics mean

An unfortunate consequence of the attention sex workers have attracted in relation to AIDS is that they tend to be seen as responsible for the spread of HIV — an attitude reflected in descriptions of prostitutes as "reservoirs of infection" or "high-frequency transmitters".

In fact, the sex worker is only the most "visible" side of a transaction that involves two people: for every sex worker who is HIV-positive there is, somewhere, the partner from whom she or he contracted the virus. And given the fact that the chance of contracting HIV during a single act of unprotected sex is not high, infection in a sex worker is likely to mean that she or he has been repeatedly exposed to the virus by clients who did not or would not wear condoms.

Thus the sound way of reading the statistics of HIV infection in sex workers is to view them as an indication of how strong a foothold the epidemic has got within a community.

in sentinel surveillance, especially to indicate the degree of HIV spread in the general population, is pregnant women attending antenatal clinics. Of course, the sentinel groups tested represent only a tiny proportion of the total number of HIV infections throughout the population, which makes the picture hard to interpret.

In sum, the shifting patterns of the epidemic, the logistic and other requirements of testing, and the need for anonymity and confidentiality make HIV/AIDS surveillance a very complex task. In many countries, surveillance activities are yet to be implemented or are only now being built up with the help of WHO (see map below). In coming years, the improved surveillance data available will begin to provide a clearer picture of the many local and regional HIV/AIDS epidemics which together make up the global epidemic.

Status of sentinel surveillance, by country, 1992

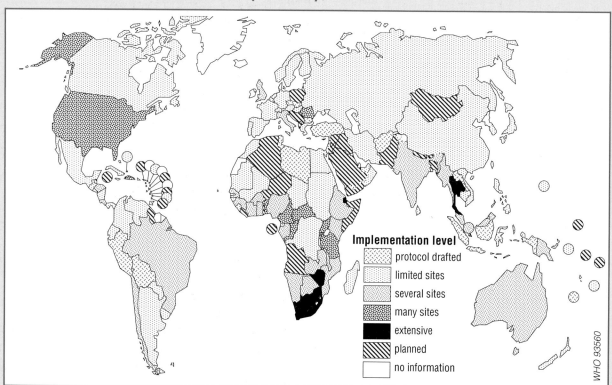

Implementation level

- protocol drafted
- limited sites
- several sites
- many sites
- extensive
- planned
- no information

WHO 93560

CHAPTER 5

Sub-Saharan Africa

In sub-Saharan Africa, one of the world's most sparsely populated areas, the epidemic spread of HIV began some 15 years ago. Therefore, not only is the HIV epidemic well advanced — the region holds a cumulative total of about 9 million infections in adults (over half of the global total) — it is also in the grip of a devastating epidemic of disease. By early 1994, according to WHO estimates, more than 2 million men, women and children in the region had become ill with AIDS. By the year 2000, the cumulative total of AIDS cases may reach 5 million.

The great majority of HIV-infected adults in sub-Saharan Africa are believed to have acquired the virus through heterosexual intercourse; and infected women outnumber men by 6 to 5. One reason appears to be the frequent presence of other STDs, which facilitate HIV transmission. Largely because of a lack of effective STD care, women in the developing world are believed to have gonorrhoea rates 10–15 times higher, and syphilis rates 10–100 times higher, than women in industrialized countries.

Close to 5 million women of childbearing age have been infected, and WHO believes that as many as 1 million children may already have been infected prior to or during birth, or through breast-feeding. This figure is expected to swell considerably by the turn of the century. Most such children have brief lives, many never know what it is to feel healthy, and some are abandoned by mothers who, ill themselves, are unable to cope with the burden of a dying child.

In this region, transmission through the transfusion of HIV-infected blood probably accounts for less than 10% of all HIV infections. Practices such as ritual scarification and the use of inadequately sterilized skin-piercing instruments are believed to account for a relatively small proportion of infections.

In nearly all areas of sub-Saharan Africa, transmission of HIV through infected blood and blood products is being reduced as appropriate screening of donated blood is introduced. Other measures being taken to protect the blood supply include recruiting donors from among low-risk population groups, on a voluntary and unpaid basis so as to discourage unsuitable donors, motivated only by money, from coming forward. Countries are also being encouraged to revise their guidelines on transfusion to ensure that the procedure is only carried out when absolutely necessary, and that saline solutions are used as blood substitutes whenever possible.

The injecting of drugs for nonmedical purposes has traditionally been a rarity in sub-Saharan Africa. However, there are indications that the practice may be catching on, particularly in port areas and among educated and affluent city-dwellers.

The area hardest hit by the epidemic is central and east Africa, which accounts for one-sixth of the region's population but between half and two-thirds of its infections. Here, in several towns and cities, a quarter or even one-third of all men and women aged 15–49 are estimated to be HIV-positive.

In 1990, the infection rate was typically far higher in urban than in rural areas. But the differential has since narrowed, and very high infection rates have been recorded in some rural areas — especially in those where good roads or navigable rivers facilitate movement to and from towns and cities.

The HIV/AIDS epidemic is now well established in west and southern Africa as well, and is thought to have travelled the trade routes with truckers and migrant workers who form liaisons away from home or have casual sex partners. Zimbabwe estimates that more than 600 000 people have been infected with HIV.

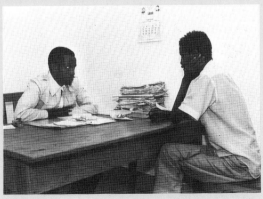

A Tanzanian man has just been told by the hospital social worker that his HIV test was positive.

In the major urban areas of Botswana, studies suggest that approximately 18% of people aged 15–49 are now infected. And in South Africa nationwide sentinel surveillance among antenatal clinic attenders indicates that the number of HIV-infected people doubled between 1990 and 1991. Sentinel surveillance data from Nigeria in early 1992 indicate extensive HIV spread in the country, with rates of 15–20% in certain groups of female prostitutes. In Abidjan, Côte d'Ivoire, where AIDS is already the leading cause of death among adults, HIV prevalence in the general population is currently thought to be 10–12%.

The spread of HIV in sub-Saharan Africa has been spurred by mass population move-

"An environment of death"

"This is an environment of death," says Protase Karani, who heads a Tanzanian home-based care team in Kagera Region on the shores of Lake Victoria. "So many people in the villages round here have died that those in the sexually active age group are frightened and unsure. Nobody is prepared to do anything very permanent."

When a man sees his wife die of AIDS and his son or daughter returns from the city also sick, why should he invest in the future? asks Karani. Why should he spend money on coffee trees that will take several years to mature, or plough more land than necessary to feed his family this year? "Today many people are spending whatever money they have on drink because they say: 'What is the point? I shall die soon too.' That's what I mean by an environment of death."

In Kasheni, a Tanzanian village bordering Lake Victoria, village chairman Gerald Ndyekobola turns the yellowed pages of a well-worn personal file in which he keeps photographs of villagers who have died. Among the portraits and snapshots of family groups is a photo of eleven fit and smiling young men who made up the local football team. More than half the figures are now marked with an ink cross indicating that they have become casualties of the epidemic.

Ndyekobola recalls a market in nearby Rukunyo, where Tanzanian and Ugandan traders did brisk business in second-hand clothing, sisal, bicycle tyres and other goods. Then people began to fall ill. When it was discovered that the sickness was AIDS, traders drifted away, the market died, and the surrounding bars and hotels gradually closed their doors.

ments due mainly to war, poverty, drought, and, some say, to poor development decisions. "The fact that HIV thrives on social unrest and poverty is clearly illustrated by the situation in this country," said Professor Nicky Padayachee, an epidemiologist in Johannesburg. Several years of violence between rival political groups in the townships and rural villages of the troubled KwaZulu-Natal province have bred a kind of fatalism, which is reflected in an unwillingness to take precautions against infection on the grounds that it will do no good. Family life and education have been disrupted as people fled their homes and the violence. One survey of more than 5000 people in the north of the province found that HIV seroprevalence — 1.2% at the end of 1990 — doubled in the next six months. It would be surprising if similarly rapid HIV spread were not occurring in war-ravaged populations across the continent, from Liberia to Zaire, Angola to Mozambique, in some cases through rape by soldiers.

Some observers believe that homosexual intercourse plays some role in HIV transmission in Africa, although homosexuality is so heavily stigmatized in this part of the world that little is known about its extent or associated behaviours. It is clear, however, that the

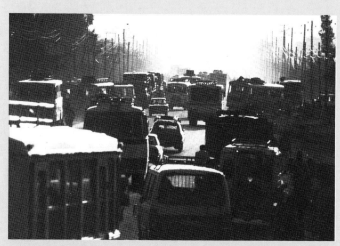

Nazareth, Ethiopia. Life on the move is not conducive to stable sex partnerships or mutual fidelity. High rates of HIV infection have been found along the main trade routes of Africa.

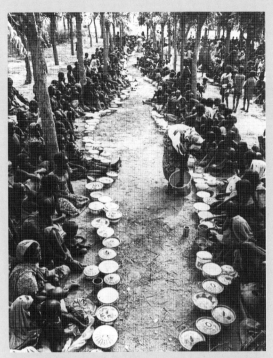

Drought in the Sahel. Natural disasters have played a part in the spread of AIDS by breaking apart community life and disrupting stable relationships.

predominant route in Africa is heterosexual intercourse.

One cause for optimism is that the rural areas of sub-Saharan Africa are still less affected by HIV/AIDS than the cities and towns, although the differential appears to be narrowing. But even in cities where HIV prevalence is high — say, 20% — it is important to bear in mind that 80% of the adult population is *not* infected. These people can still avert infection if the right information and services get to them in time. Another cause for optimism is that in many countries close to half the population is under 15 years old and in many cases not yet sexually active. If effective AIDS education campaigns are developed for youngsters, there are grounds for hope that the next generation will not be so badly hit by this disease.

CHAPTER 6

South and south-east Asia

WHO believes that if effective HIV prevention programmes are not put in place, Asia will overtake Africa by the mid to late 1990s in terms of the number of newly infected people per year. Asia is a decade or so behind Africa, but HIV transmission rates in some population groups in south and south-east Asia today are as high as they were 10 years ago in sub-Saharan Africa. And because of the difference in population sizes, what is happening in Africa now could be dwarfed by the Asian epidemic.

Fortunately, HIV rates in the general population are still relatively low even in the worst-affected countries of this region. Asia thus has a chance to avert catastrophe that Africa — hit by the epidemic before anyone knew anything about HIV — did not have.

WHO estimates that more than 2 million adults have been infected to date. Most infections thus far are thought to have been in India, Thailand and Myanmar, but the virus is spreading quickly among vulnerable groups elsewhere.

Because epidemic HIV spread in this part of the world did not begin until the late 1980s, there had been only an estimated 30 000 AIDS cases by mid-1993, but WHO projects that this figure will rise to 1.4 million by the end of the century.

For the region's adults, the predominant modes of transmission are unprotected heterosexual intercourse and needle-sharing. Homosexual transmission is also thought to play some role in the region, although it is difficult to quantify because this form of sexuality is often hidden.

In India, an indication of the population's vulnerability to HIV can be found in the millions of STDs occurring each year. In addition to being a "marker" for behavioural vulnerability to HIV infection, untreated STDs facilitate HIV transmission. In Pune, a city near Bombay, HIV infection rates among people seeking STD care climbed from nearly 9% in 1991 to 17% in 1992. Infection rates of up to 25% were reported in 1992 from surveys among prostitutes in Bombay.

In Myanmar, surveys among STD patients have found a steep rise in the prevalence of HIV infection, the rates rising from close to zero in 1989 to around 8% by 1991. Such a rise demon-

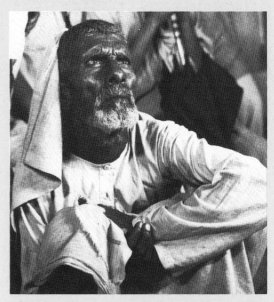

In most of the world there is no formal social security — people expect to be supported in their old age by their adult sons and daughters. But because of AIDS, elderly people will be left without support — and many may find themselves burdened with the care of orphaned grandchildren.

strates how explosive the spread of HIV can be once it gains a foothold in a population, especially where condom use is low. In 1991, in Thailand, where HIV infection rates of 10-20% have been seen among men seeking care at STD clinics, one survey found that about half of Thai men questioned said they never used condoms.

In some Asian countries, a large proportion of sex outside marriage is not "casual sex" but "commercial sex", i.e. sex in exchange for money. "When a boy in the Western world goes on his first date, many boys in Thailand visit their first female prostitute", says Mr Mechai Viravaidya, Director of the Population Development Association and a leading anti-AIDS campaigner. One study found that 44% of Thai men had their first sexual experience with a prostitute at an average age of about 18 years. Figures from the Royal Thai Army, Armed Forces Research Institute of Medical Sciences, show that new recruits to the army in 1992 had an HIV prevalence of 3.7% for the country as a whole, up from 2% in 1990. Among 21–23 year olds from the far north, prevalence was 14–19% on recruitment in November 1991; 9 months later, a further 3.9% of the uninfected recruits had become HIV-positive.

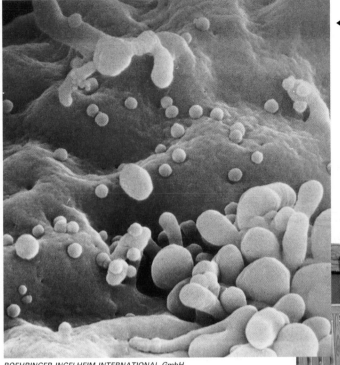

Portrait of a virus, magnified about 30 000 times. On the mountain-like surface of a T lymphocyte infected by HIV, the virus particles are seen as small, rounded or hexagonal dots.

AIDS orphans and babies abandoned by HIV-positive mothers who fear they may have passed on the infection to their offspring are a tragic feature of the epidemic almost everywhere. In this photo from Poland, the children are cared for in an orphanage.

▼

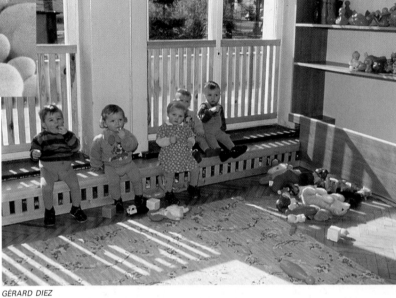

A Masai woman sells traditional medicine in Dar es Salaam's central market. In many countries, traditional healers are the first, and sometimes the only, resort when people are sick. They can be valuable allies in the fight against AIDS.

▼

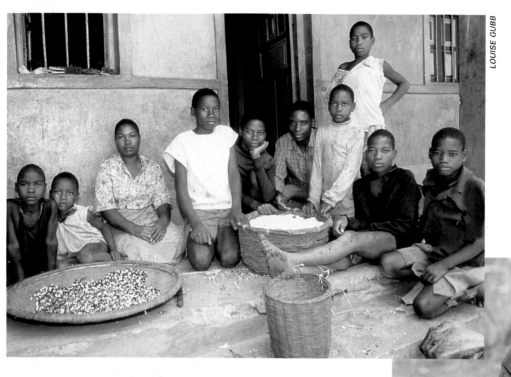

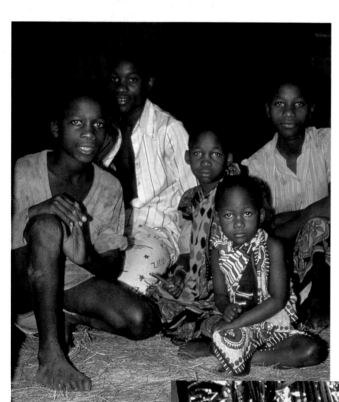

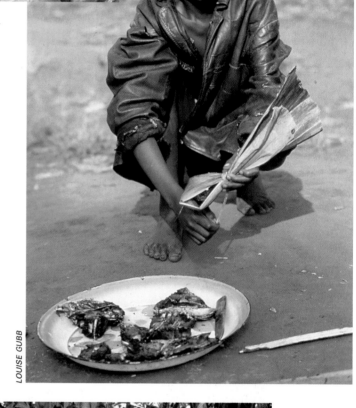

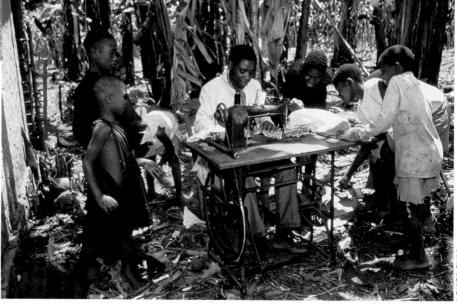

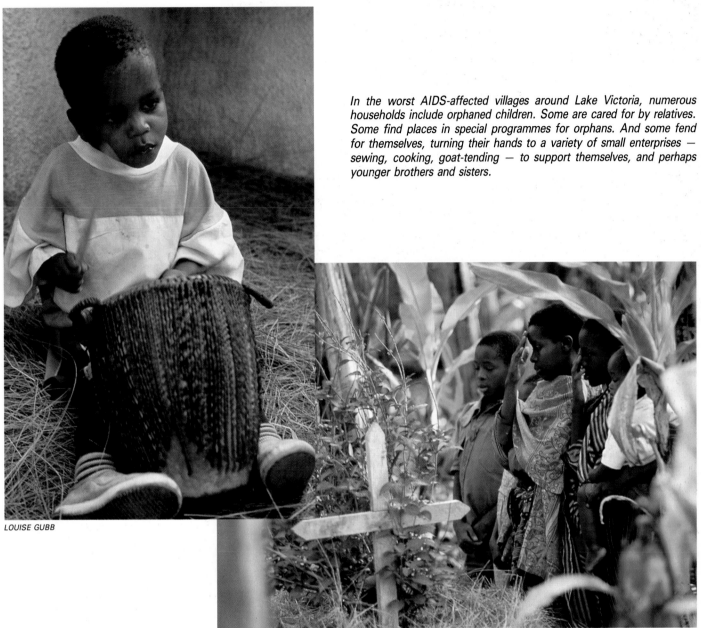

In the worst AIDS-affected villages around Lake Victoria, numerous households include orphaned children. Some are cared for by relatives. Some find places in special programmes for orphans. And some fend for themselves, turning their hands to a variety of small enterprises — sewing, cooking, goat-tending — to support themselves, and perhaps younger brothers and sisters.

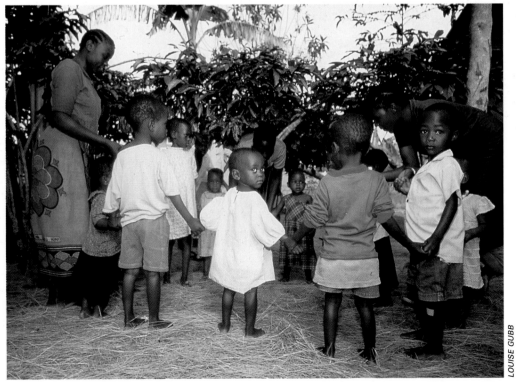

◀ *Over a period of just two years, this man watched seven members of his family, including a small grandchild, die in the epidemic. The months of hopeless nursing haunt his memory and he has given up the will to live though he himself does not have AIDS.*

Young hill-tribe women in Thailand.
▼

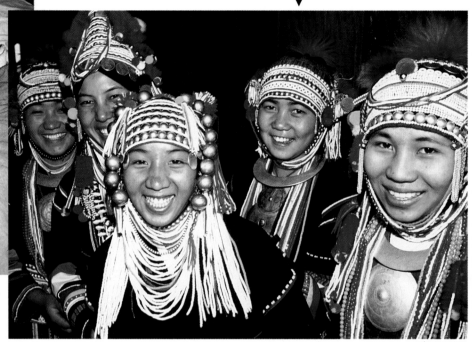

LOUISE GUBB

GÉRARD DIEZ

In this rural Tanzanian market, practically anything can be bought but condoms. A multitude of logistic problems have interrupted condom supplies, making it hard for people in this region of high HIV prevalence to protect themselves from infection.
▼

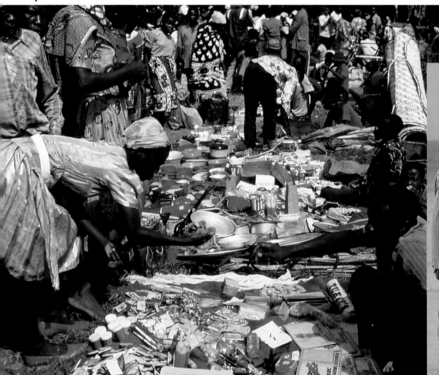

LOUISE GUBB

In the United Republic of Tanzania, the condition that later became ▶ known as AIDS was dubbed "hella's disease" ("the disease of money") in 1981 because the people most affected by it seemed to be prosperous fishermen and merchants trading around Lake Victoria.

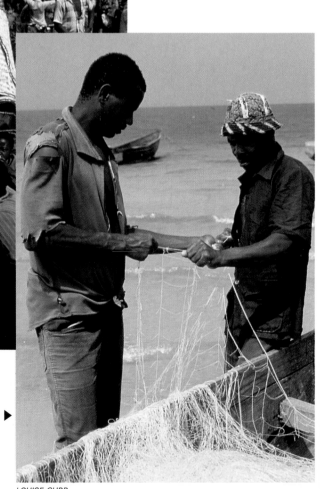

LOUISE GUBB

Once high levels of infection have been found among sex workers and clients, it is only a matter of time before people outside these particularly vulnerable groups are drawn into the circle of infection. Among pregnant Thai women attending antenatal clinics, for example, HIV prevalence has reached 4% in at least five provinces. As Jon Ungphakorn, director of the AIDS Counselling Centre Educational Support Service (ACCESS), has observed of his country: "For married women it has become high-risk behaviour to have unprotected sex with their husbands, unless they are absolutely certain that their husbands are not visiting sex establishments" (9).

The AIDS epidemic in south and southeast Asia gained an early foothold among injecting drug users in the region, and they remain hard-hit today. People who inject drugs are by no means a homogeneous group. In many cities, drug use tends to be associated with poverty and crime, as it is in industrialized countries. In countries with a long tradition of opium-smoking, however, this kind of drug use is comparable to alcohol use elsewhere, especially among older people.

In recent years, however, the region's drug scene has begun to change. While older people have tended to smoke opium, younger people begin their drug use smoking heroin, a derivative of opium, and eventually start injecting the drug in order to increase its effect. As communities began to experience the grim effects of this variation of the habit, older social tolerance gave way to condemnation and rejection. These attitudes have become even more pronounced since the emergence of AIDS. Reports have come from a number of places of drug users being summarily imprisoned, or confined in "rehabilitation centres" resembling prison camps, or even attacked and beaten to death in the streets. Even milder forms of stigmatization are hampering efforts to bring the HIV epidemic under control. For instance, it is hard for health authorities to follow up on drug users who are HIV-positive because visiting their homes can bring shame on their families and ostracism by friends and neighbours.

Today the virus is spreading rapidly in and around the area known as the Golden Triangle, where the territories of the Lao People's Democratic Republic, Myanmar and Thailand meet, and where most of the world's opium and heroin are produced.

In Myanmar, there has been a steep rise in infection rates fuelled by poverty and by strict action against drug-taking. Needles and syringes are expensive, so many people improvise injecting equipment which they then share; or they have their drugs injected by dealers, who use the same needles and syringes on many clients. The sharing of injection equipment is also encouraged by the fact that possession of needles and syringes — by anyone other than a health professional or a diabetic — is used by police as evidence of drug-taking, which is strictly punishable by law. Needle-sharing is practised, too, out of camaraderie.

Like Myanmar, India has been drawn into the drugs and AIDS vortex of the Golden Triangle and it provides a clear example of the dynamics of the epidemic among drug users. Heroin use became established among the people of the north-eastern State of Manipur, which borders Myanmar, around 1984 and the practice of injecting the drug was soon widespread among users. Research by India's National Institute for Cholera and Enteric Diseases suggests that there are around 15 000 – 20 000 injecting drug users in the State out of a total population of 1.8 million. Initially middle-class, well educated youngsters, Manipur's drug users are increasingly found in all strata of society, as they tend to be elsewhere in India, for example, in Nagaland, bordering Manipur to the north.

In Thailand, where infection rates among injecting drug users are rising steeply, heroin use is implicated in the spread of HIV not only directly through the sharing of needles, but also indirectly through complex links with sex work. Young village women are recruited by visiting middle-men who claim to be offering jobs in restaurants, teashops or private homes but who are really recruiting for the sex industry. In some cases, families agree to allow their daughters to work off loans (debt bondage), and in some cases they "sell" their daughters outright.

From some hill tribes, one in five young women is drawn into prostitution, according to the Chiang Mai Hill Tribes Welfare and

People living in Shan State, Myanmar (formerly Burma), were familiar with AIDS several years before it was recognized by their government. It was known as "dangerous disease coming from outside".

Development Centre. In some cases, the recruits are imprisoned by the brothel-owners during their initiation into the business. Such stories are rarely told in the villages, however, for the young women who return home dressed in modern clothes and make-up are too proud to relate the price they have had to pay for this superficial glamour and for the survival of their families.

Extremely high rates of HIV infection have been reported among such women, who are especially vulnerable because most are illiterate and speak no Thai — and little effort is made to reach them with AIDS information. They also tend to work in the lowest-class brothels catering for local Thai men, where they have 5 – 10 clients a night at a rate of around US$1 – 2 each — a sum shared between the prostitute and the brothel-owner.

Apart from unprotected sex and drug injection, contaminated blood transfusions are thought to contribute to the epidemic in parts of south and south-east Asia. In India, the trading of blood for transfusion and the preparation of blood products is big business and subject to very little control. Infection rates among donors vary but generally are higher among professional donors than among voluntary donors, who give blood without remuneration.

Blood screening facilities are in general available only in major cities, and in 1989 – 90 it was estimated that less than 30% of donated blood was screened for HIV, although the goal is to screen more than 60 – 70% of blood by 1994. To try to minimize the risk of transmitting the virus through blood transfusions, the Ministry of Health and the Indian Council of Medical Research have an official policy not to use blood procured from the open market (i.e. from paid blood donors) in government health services.

The experiences of India, Myanmar and Thailand could easily be repeated in other countries of the region — particularly Bangladesh, Indonesia, Malaysia, Nepal and Sri Lanka, where illicit drug injection, high STD rates, male patronage of female and male prostitutes, and/or low rates of condom usage in both casual and long-term relationships are common. Countries such as Cambodia, the Lao People's Democratic Republic and Viet Nam, which are emerging from the isolating influence of communism, are also especially vulnerable to HIV infection as their people go through profound social and economic changes. It is therefore vital that education, condom promotion and community action programmes are put in place throughout the region.

CHAPTER 7

East Asia and the Pacific

The enormous diversity of cultures, political systems and socioeconomic conditions in East Asia and the Pacific is paralleled by the wide range of patterns of HIV infection in this region where HIV began to spread in the mid-1980s.

As of early 1994, WHO estimates that the region as a whole had more than 25 000 infections in adults. Japan estimates that the cumulative total in that country was around 11 000 at the end of 1992, up from some 8000 one year earlier.

Fewer than 1000 AIDS cases have been reported to date from the region. Japan has reported the highest number: a total of 566 as of April 1993. But other smaller islands — notably French Polynesia, New Caledonia and Guam — have a higher rate of AIDS per 100 000 population.

In Japan, most cases thus far have been in men with haemophilia reported to have received contaminated factor VIII, and HIV infections have been found in people with haemophilia in Hong Kong and China (Province of Taiwan) as well. These commercial products were usually prepared from what is known as "source plasma" obtained from paid donors, prior to the availability of HIV testing and, more recently, viral inactivation procedures. Transmission through blood transfusions has been minimal, as HIV testing of blood for transfusion was introduced at the same time as in most developed countries. Around 1990 the rate of heterosexual infections in Japan began to rise dramatically, marking the beginning of a new trend in the pattern of HIV transmission in that country. Whereas in 1990 under half of all reported HIV infections and AIDS cases in Japan were in women, by 1992 women outnumbered men by about three to two.

AIDS in Hong Kong has affected mainly homosexual and bisexual men. In French Polynesia, too, more than half of all cases have been in men who have sex with men, while more than 20% have been linked to heterosexual transmission. In Papua New Guinea, more than half of all HIV infections have been transmitted heterosexually.

As in much of the world, STDs were not high on the public health agenda before the advent of AIDS, and information on STD rates — which would give an indication of the population's vulnerability to HIV infection — is inconsistent and unreliable. From preliminary data from Papua New Guinea, Fiji and elsewhere in the South Pacific, it appears that certain STDs are more common than was once believed. In Papua New Guinea, for example, limited studies in women attending antenatal clinics indicate that between 11% and 22% have chlamydia infection.

Very few cases of AIDS have been reported from the vast territory and population of China, though serological surveys indicate that HIV has taken root among injecting drug users in the south-western province of Yunnan, which shares a border with Myanmar in the Golden Triangle area. The numbers of people involved in injecting drug use, which is illegal, highly stigmatized and therefore secretive, are unknown. But infection rates of 10–35% among drug injectors were recorded in 1990. Most affected are minority groups living in the mountains close to the China/Myanmar border, which people cross freely for personal visits or to trade with neighbouring villages. Drug use in this area is predominantly a male habit.

A number of demographic and economic features could well affect the dynamics of the HIV/AIDS epidemic in this region: its immense population size, its population density (far greater than that in Africa or Latin America), and its booming urban economies leading to huge population shifts from rural to urban areas, fuelled by hopes of greater economic opportunities. On the plus side, half a century of investment in education has left much of Asia literate and hence easy to reach with information on AIDS; many rural people have access to television and other media; and family planning programmes have been established for nearly 30 years, providing a good infrastructure for condom distribution and STD care. Where condoms are already a popular family planning method, the challenge is to persuade men to see them as effective tools for disease prevention too, and to use them above all for casual sex —the behaviour through which HIV is now spreading so rapidly.

CHAPTER 8

Latin America and the Caribbean

In Latin America and the Caribbean, where WHO estimates that there have already been about 1.5 million HIV infections in adults, the virus has been spreading extensively since the late 1970s or early 1980s. As in Western Europe and the USA, the epidemic arose mainly in big cities among homosexual and bisexual men, among injecting drug users and, to a lesser extent, among recipients of commercially supplied blood and blood products. But since the mid to late 1980s heterosexual transmission has increased steadily, principally between bisexual men and their female sex partners, between male and female drug injectors and their sex partners, between female sex workers and their male clients, and between the latter and their regular partners.

Thus far, there have been about a quarter of a million AIDS cases in adults and children in this region. Brazil, whose population of around 150 million makes it the fourth largest country in the world, has the highest number of reported AIDS cases in the Americas, after the USA — 40 000. As of December 1992, Colombia and Venezuela together had reported over 5000 cumulative AIDS cases, and Argentina over 2000 cases. The rate of reported AIDS cases per 100 000 population was 5.6 in 1991 in Brazil, but far higher rates were observed in some Caribbean islands where the population is much smaller.

In Brazil, heterosexual transmission — linked to only 7.5% of reported AIDS cases up to 1987 — accounted for 23% by 1992. Primarily for this reason, women are increasingly affected: the male/female ratio was 28 to 1 in 1985 and only 5 to 1 in 1992. Studies among pregnant women attending antenatal clinics in São Paulo state between 1987 and 1990 found that seroprevalence increased steadily during the period, from 0.2% to 1.3%.

The situation in Central America is also causing concern. In 1991, 0.6% of male police employees in Guatemala City were found to be infected. Meanwhile, in San Pedro Sula, Honduras, studies in pregnant women conducted in 1991 revealed infection rates of 3.6%. In a nearby commune close to the Guatemalan border, a 1992 HIV prevalence study of sex workers, whose clients are mostly truck drivers, found around one-third to be infected. Around 10% of STD clinic attenders in Honduras were also infected with HIV, reflecting the close epidemiological link between HIV infection and the conventional STDs.

In the Caribbean, which has some of the highest per capita AIDS rates in the world, heterosexual intercourse is the main mode of HIV transmission. And AIDS is occurring in ever-younger people. The Caribbean Epidemiology Center reports that young people between 15 and 29 now account for more than 50% of all AIDS cases — up from 30% in 1986. Many are thus infected with HIV as teenagers.

Elsewhere, too, young people are at risk. In a survey in Rio de Janeiro, some 44% of men aged 15–49 reported engaging in sexual intercourse outside a regular partnership. But among young men aged 15–19, the proportion was around 60%. Rates as high as this were not seen among similar samples of male teenagers surveyed in other parts of the world.

An important early factor in the spread of HIV in some areas of South America was the number of men whose primary relationships were with women but who also had sex with other men. For example, a study of women diagnosed with AIDS in Mexico up to December 1990 showed that, of those for whom information was available about their sex partner, 46% had a bisexual partner.

In many parts of Latin America, as elsewhere in the world, men are by tradition permitted to seek sex prior to and outside of marriage, while women are expected to remain virgins before marriage and monogamous thereafter. A study in Mexico observes that it is socially acceptable for men to have sex with a homosexual partner provided they take the active, insertive role in anal intercourse — a role regarded as "macho", i.e. super-masculine. The same-sex partner may be a boy who sells sex occasionally for the price of a new shirt or pair of shoes. In Peru, where more than half a million children under the age of 14 live in families struggling below the poverty line, this form of occasional prostitution is known as *fleteo*. Or the relationship can take the form of sex barter whereby, as has been observed in Mexico, apprentices in the construction trade may be afforded some degree of protection (e.g. job stability) in exchange for sex.

In some parts of Latin America, HIV transmission through needle-sharing is causing special alarm. In Brazil, the proportion of reported AIDS patients who injected drugs rose dramatically between 1986 and 1991. One of the worst affected cities is Santos, the port city of São Paulo, which bustles with shipping traffic, trade and tourism. The injecting of cocaine — especially dangerous because it may involve 5 – 6 injections a day — is said to be reaching epidemic proportions, and serosurveys in Santos have found rates of HIV infection of 50 – 60% among users.

While sexual exposure to bisexual men and to male or female drug users accounted for a significant proportion of HIV infections among heterosexuals early in the epidemic, today their overwhelming risk factor is exposure to another heterosexual. This is especially true where heterosexual transmission is spurred by a high prevalence of STDs and other genital tract infections, due to inadequate access to early detection and treatment, and by poverty and social misery which favour unprotected sex with many partners, frequently as part of a strategy of survival through sex work. If AIDS prevention is to be successful, strategies must be found for confronting or circumventing these conditions, for they exist to varying degrees in practically every country of the region.

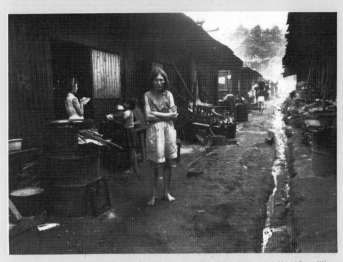

A refugee camp in Central America. Life for the world's 18 million refugees is harsh and uncertain. Many live without the most basic facilities, beyond the reach of education, information, health care and commodities. Most are women and children. They are powerless, open to sexual abuse, and especially vulnerable to HIV infection.

CHAPTER 9

Australasia, north America and western Europe

By WHO's estimates, the industrialized countries of Australasia, north America and western Europe, where extensive HIV spread began in the late 1970s to early 1980s, have had more than 1.5 million infections in adults. Over 1 million of these are estimated to be in the USA.

The USA has by far the highest reported rate of AIDS in the industrialized world, with a cumulative total of 114 cases per 100 000 population by end 1992. (Spain and France, second and third in the industrialized world, had reported 44 and 40 cases per 100 000 respectively by the same date.) By the end of the 1980s the epidemic had already claimed more American lives than the Korean and Viet Nam wars put together.

The first identified cases of AIDS appeared in the USA among homosexual and bisexual men, injecting drug users, and recipients of blood products. Homosexual/bisexual men and injecting drug users still account for the majority of AIDS cases in industrialized countries as a whole, but heterosexual transmission, especially to women, is increasing fast in certain communities.

Studies show how HIV moved rapidly through the gay communities of San Francisco and New York before anyone knew there was a new disease called AIDS. From 1978 onwards, the San Francisco City Clinic, specializing in STDs, collected blood samples from homosexual and bisexual men taking part in a research project on hepatitis B. In 1985, when it became possible to detect HIV in the blood, the frozen and stored samples from 746 of the men were tested for the virus and the same men agreed to further tests. Mathematical modelling based on the data suggested that 6% of the men had been infected with HIV in 1978, 19% in 1979, and 33% in 1980. By 1985, 70% had been infected. Today, HIV transmission through sex between men accounts for nine-tenths of cumulative AIDS cases on the west coast of the USA and two-fifths on the east coast.

In Australia the vast majority of AIDS cases have been due to homosexual transmission. The worst affected state is New South Wales, where Sydney, the state capital, has long

> "An unplanned outcome of the gay liberation movement of the 1970s," write Ron Stall and Jay Paul, "was a vast business of gay bathhouses and sex clubs. These establishments capitalized on the prevailing ethos, in which pressing beyond the limits of conventional sexual behaviour was a political act, proof positive of one's freedom from repressive social norms. At the same time, this institutionalization or commercialization of sex led to a tremendous increase in sexually transmitted diseases, which the most sexually active of this population treated as a routine and expected result of sexual activity that was readily treatable by the medical establishment" (10).

had a large homosexual community. Although the city's residents make up just over a fifth of Australia's population, they accounted for well over half its reported AIDS cases in early 1991.

In the Nordic countries — Denmark, Finland, Iceland, Norway and Sweden — homosexual transmission of HIV accounted for

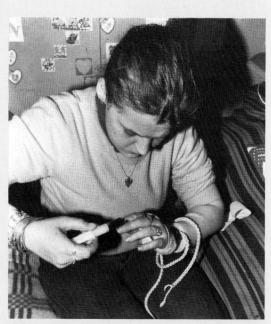

In some parts of the developed world, injecting drug users are the population group most affected by HIV/AIDS.

between 61% and 74% of cumulative AIDS cases by early 1993, compared with a maximum of 12% through needle-sharing by drug users. This is in marked contrast to the countries of southern Europe, where AIDS affects mainly drug injectors. In Italy and mainland Spain, injecting drug users constitute almost two-thirds of AIDS cases. Serosurveys among certain groups of injectors have found HIV infection rates of up to 58% in France, 30 – 80% in Italy, and 40 – 60% in Spain. Around two-fifths of all AIDS cases in Ireland and Switzerland are due to needle-sharing. In the USA, nearly one-quarter of AIDS cases reported in 1992 were related to drug injecting.

In certain cities in Europe, the sharing of injection equipment is at the root of a local AIDS crisis that is in marked contrast to the picture in the country as a whole. This distinct local pattern is evident in Edinburgh, where the epidemic is centred on impoverished public housing estates on the outskirts of Scotland's otherwise prosperous capital (see panel).

The incidence of infection among homosexual men is falling. Having witnessed the slow, painful deaths of so many friends and partners in the earliest years of the epidemic — and often the inaction of the authorities — gay men were the first to take up the challenge of AIDS. They have had remarkable successes in reducing risk behaviour.

However, there is a rising tide of infections transmitted through unprotected intercourse between men and women. In western Europe overall, the proportion of AIDS cases due to heterosexual transmission has risen to more than 10%. In Finland, Norway and Switzerland, the percentage is now around 15%, and in Greece and Portugal it is 20% and 27%, respectively. In the USA, WHO estimated at the end of 1991 that about 100 000 people had been infected heterosexually.

It is not surprising, given this trend, that the number of women with HIV infection and AIDS is rising everywhere in the developed world. AIDS is now the leading cause of death among 25 – 44-year-old women in nine major US cities. In 1992, HIV prevalence among pregnant women in London ranged between 1 and 5 per 1000.

The trend towards heterosexual transmission of HIV is most marked in cities with significant populations of injecting drug users, whose high-risk behaviour increases the vulner-

Edinburgh's AIDS crisis

Muirhouse estate, on the mouth of the river Forth, is an area of chronic unemployment on the western edge of Edinburgh. In the early 1980s, when a plentiful supply of heroin began entering the city through the port of Leith, many bored and demoralized youngsters started injecting the drug. Throughout the 1970s, police believe, there were only about 40 – 50 heroin users in the region of Lothian, which includes Edinburgh. By 1983, the figure had swollen to around 2000.

In 1982 an epidemic of hepatitis B broke out among injecting drug users in Muirhouse, and some local doctors — already very involved with the drug-using community — began routine blood testing. In 1985, they tested samples of the stored blood for HIV and found that 51% proved positive — a rate more than 10 times higher than in nearby Glasgow, which had a much more established drug scene.

Local experts believe a number of factors coincided to create ideal conditions in Edinburgh for an explosive spread of HIV, starting in 1983. In an attempt to stamp out the wave of drug use, Edinburgh police had closed down the local, legal supplier of needles and syringes. Other pharmacies reacted by imposing a voluntary ban on such sales. The result: an acute shortage of injection equipment and the consequent widespread sharing of needles and syringes in the early 1980s. Furthermore, because possession of injection equipment was regarded as incriminating evidence, many people borrowed the needles and syringes of others when injecting. The intense police activity had the effect of driving drug use underground rather than curtailing it. Those affected — who tended to be young, naive and ignorant of the dangers of injecting — had little contact with health or social services. In this climate of social, medical and legal alienation, the health risks were amplified. In Glasgow, needles and syringes were not so difficult to obtain — which most observers believe is a major factor in its much lower HIV rates.

Behaviour has changed as AIDS awareness has grown, and new infections among drug users in Edinburgh are now occurring at much the same rate as in nearby Glasgow — below 2% annually. But the full effects of the 1983 – 84 epidemic are only starting to be felt in Edinburgh. Many who were teenagers when they started injecting are today married with children. In some cases, both parents are infected and their children will be orphaned. Dr Roy Robertson of the Muirhouse Medical Group practice says he is seeing more and more HIV-infected patients with obvious signs of disease. And the community is coming under growing strain as the disaster they tried to deny becomes reality. "People were able to suppress [thoughts of AIDS] but now they see their friends falling ill and are getting ill themselves. There is a level of panic building up."

In 1981, fewer than 100 people died in the USA of what came to be known as AIDS. According to the US Centers for Disease Control, by the end of 1993 there will have been 285 000 to 340 000 deaths, most of them among the homosexual men and injecting drug users who became infected ten or more years ago. And as the decade wears on, AIDS will increasingly be claiming the lives of Americans infected hetero-sexually.

"It is likely that in three or four years every American will know someone who has AIDS," Dr Michael S. Gott-lieb, who treated some of the earliest AIDS cases, wrote in *The New York Times* back in June 1991. "Maybe that is what it will take to change attitudes and make all Americans activists."

ability of their sex partners. Dr Roy Robertson of the Muirhouse Medical Group in Edinburgh regularly sees teenage girls who have contract-ed HIV through sexual intercourse. "Most often they come in with seroconversion illness and they're shocked and devastated to discover that they are HIV-positive. They'd never imagined they were doing anything risky."

This is what Robertson predicted in a report for the Scottish health department in 1989, when he said that, although the num-bers shown to be infected heterosexually were still small, there was no room for complacen-cy. "The experience in Scotland closely parallels that in northern Italy, where heterosexual cases are now emerging rapidly a few years after the caseload of infected intravenous drug misusers."

There are often direct links between drug use and prostitution, as some drug users sell sex to support their habit. Many of the female prostitutes who frequent a drop-in centre in Glasgow's "red light" district are injecting drug users. Since they are desperate to earn money to pay for the drug, they do not always ask for — or obtain — condom use by their clients. At least one study has found that many clients look for women who use drugs precisely in order to avoid having to use a condom.

WHO's projections suggest that although HIV is unlikely to spread explosively in the industrialized world as it is in Africa and Asia, people will continue to get infected throughout this decade. Young homosexual men and poor city-dwelling heterosexuals with high rates of STDs and drug injecting are par-ticularly vulnerable. Keeping the rate of new infections low will require constant education and community organization to encourage and support safer behaviour.

At best, because of the long lag between initial infection with HIV and the development of AIDS, it must be borne in mind that the crisis for industrialized countries will not end even if new infections slow down dramatical-ly. WHO projects that cumulative AIDS deaths by the year 2000 will be triple what they are today.

CHAPTER 10

North Africa, the Horn of Africa and the eastern Mediterranean area

This region presents at least two epidemiological pictures. In some communities, notably in the Horn of Africa and southern Sudan, the pattern of HIV transmission is similar to that in sub-Saharan Africa. In other parts of the region, the epidemic is not well documented and only limited information is available about the routes or magnitude of transmission.

Worst affected thus far are the huge territories of Ethiopia and Sudan, parts of the Maghreb, and Djibouti. The first International Arab Conference on AIDS held in Egypt in March 1988 marked the acknowledgement by many countries in the region that risk factors seen elsewhere in the world — social instability and poverty, commercial sex, drug injecting and homosexual behaviour between men — exist in their populations, and that the mobility of people in a region where so many migrate in search of work or education means that no country can be isolated from the threat.

As of mid-1993, fewer than 1400 AIDS cases had been reported to WHO, with only one country reporting no cases. Given the considerable under-recognition and under-reporting in many countries, the actual number of cases is considered to be much higher. Of the reported cases, 75% are in males and 25% in females, the majority due to sexual transmission. WHO

estimates that a cumulative total of more than 75 000 adults had become infected by early 1994.

A thriving sex industry has established itself around the busy Red Sea port of Djibouti, as women fleeing crippling poverty and war in neighbouring countries have seen a chance to make a living. According to Djibouti's national AIDS programme, the clients of street prostitutes tend to be local men, while the bar girls cater for foreign sailors and military men and the local elite. As the programme reported in January 1993, HIV infection rates of 51% have been found among street prostitutes, 22% among bar girls, and 12% among men attending STD clinics. Infection rates in Djibouti are now rising too among people not especially associated with high-risk behaviour.

In southern Sudan, where civil war has displaced much of the population, the HIV/AIDS problem continues to grow. The number of AIDS cases reported in 1991 was 40% higher than the year before. Heterosexual intercourse was reported in 1991 as being the route of transmission behind 94% of cases. In southern Sudan relationships between the sexes are traditionally less circumscribed than in the Muslim north, but even in some northern population groups premarital sex may be condoned as a means of testing the fertility of girls and increasing the population.

In the northern city of Khartoum, the Sudanese capital, where all donated blood is screened, the proportion of HIV-infected samples increased tenfold between 1987 and late 1992.

Though efforts are being made to ensure safe blood supplies in major hospitals throughout Sudan, chronic shortages of facilities, equipment and materials mean that only about 30% of donated blood is screened for HIV. Tests conducted before 1990 on 33 recipients of blood found that 16 had contracted the virus. Varying levels of transmission through contaminated blood have been also been reported in Algeria, Egypt, Libyan Arab Jamahirya, Islamic Republic of Iran, and Tunisia.

Ethiopia, which shares a long border and many social problems with Sudan, is particularly open about its epidemic. "We have here

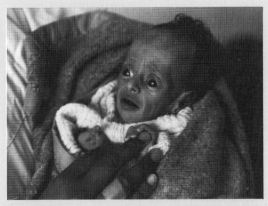

Whereas most illnesses produce sympathy and support from family, friends and neighbours, AIDS often elicits irrational fear and withdrawal. Here, an abandoned HIV-infected baby is cared for in a home in Addis Ababa.

the same preconditions for a rapid spread of AIDS as existed in Uganda: civil war, the displacement of people, a deteriorating economy,'' says Dr Mekonnen Bishaw, head of social science at Addis Ababa University. "All the conditions exist for an explosion of HIV infection, and it's very worrying.''

By the end of 1991, Ethiopia had reported 1631 cases of AIDS. But serosurveys in urban centres have found extremely high levels of HIV infection in certain population groups, and by 1993 the Ministry of Health was using a working estimate of close to half a million infections.

The worst-affected population groups in Ethiopia, which has a population of around 50 million, are female prostitutes and their clients. At least 200 000 women are estimated to survive through prostitution, most of them from northern rural areas where poverty, war, drought and famine have driven many from the land. The majority are poorly educated and unskilled, but even educated women are turning up in bars and brothels as the economy deteriorates.

Members of the armed forces accounted for 17% of the AIDS cases reported in Ethiopia up to 1991, twice the proportion accounted for by female prostitutes. The national AIDS programme fears that infection rates will rise sharply in rural areas — where the bulk of Ethiopia's population lives — as soldiers from what was Africa's biggest army return home, after the long civil war, to become farmers.

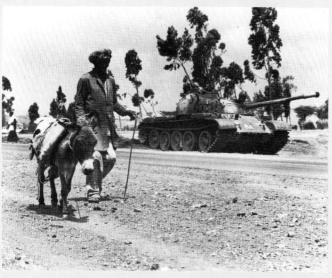

The social breakdown that accompanies war creates ideal conditions for the spread of HIV. In Ethiopia, the countryside is still littered with the relics of the 17-year civil war that helped fuel one of the worst AIDS epidemics in the region.

Among long-distance lorry drivers, HIV infection rates of 15 – 20% were reached as long ago as 1990. Most drivers travel the main road between Addis Ababa and the port city of Assab, now in Eritrea. Cases of AIDS and HIV infection are clustered all along this route in towns full of hotels and bars catering for a highly mobile population of merchants, businessmen and other travellers.

The administration of injections by unqualified health practitioners may also be contributing to HIV transmission. Ethiopian people, especially rural people, believe injections to be more effective than tablets, says Dr Hailu Negassa of the Department of AIDS Control. Many community health agents or traditional birth attendants — or even just cleaners at hospitals who have access to supplies of needles and syringes — have set up private clinics to exploit this belief. "These people are accepted by their communities and we think it is a problem,'' says Negassa.

Injecting drug use plays a role in the spread of HIV in the Maghreb countries of North Africa, which have strong historic and economic links with Europe. In Tunisia, for example, needle-sharing accounted for around three-quarters of AIDS cases to 1992, most of which have reportedly occurred among Tunisians who travelled to Europe for work or study. Very little information is available on AIDS in Mauritania, but there are thought to be many drug users at high risk of infection. An HIV prevalence of about 14% was reported among injecting drug users known to police authorities in one Gulf state in 1989.

The preponderance of men among injecting drug users helps explain why, among the region's AIDS cases, men outnumber women. Unprotected sex between men is another factor. However, in parts of the world where homosexual and bisexual behaviour is condemned, it is important to obtain information about this transmission route in a useful way. Pressuring men with HIV infection to admit they had sex with men is not only unethical — it interferes with AIDS prevention and endangers the public health.

Of the approximately 1500 HIV infections among resident and immigrant expatriates reported over the past seven years in one Gulf state, one-third were believed to have occurred during 1992 alone, indicating the rapid evolution of the epidemic in the region.

Although some countries of the region still assert that AIDS will never be a major problem for them because the cultural and moral values of their societies are not conducive to the spread of HIV, many countries now show great willingness and determination to confront the epidemic. A positive sign is that religious leaders have become more involved in the response to AIDS, and many advocate a compassionate attitude towards people with the disease. It is also encouraging that where religious and cultural sensibilities limit frank discussion about sexuality and make it difficult for officials to promote condoms, independent, nongovernmental groups have sprung up to take action.

Sex work and begging

Berhane, a fragile woman in her mid-twenties, works in a bar in Nazareth, Ethiopia, serving "tej" — a thick yellow alcoholic drink made from honey. She was married at the age of nine. After her children died at the ages of four and two, she fled rural poverty and an abusive husband for the city, where work as a barmaid was all she could find. As the bar owner gives only board and lodging in return for her work, cash has to be earned through prostitution. "This life is not much better than what I ran away from, but what can I do?" she says. "At least it's better than begging."

Almaz also chose sex work as the only alternative to begging. Moving from the north to live with relatives in Addis Ababa on the death of her parents, she had to drop out of school when her aunt there died. She works at the lower end of the sex industry in a "red light" — a tiny rented room which is also her home. All along the narrow alleyway, doors open on similar dingy rooms. Outside, young women in colourful dresses chat, comb their hair, lean against the door-jambs and wait for clients.

CHAPTER 11

Eastern Europe and central Asia

Information from this region, which includes countries of the former Soviet Union, indicates that its epidemic is about five years behind that in western Europe. Only Hungary, Romania and Slovenia have reported more than one AIDS case per 100 000 population. However, the epidemic is growing. For the region as a whole, WHO estimates that more than 50 000 adults have already been infected with HIV.

As the result of an outbreak in Romania, around 2000 children were infected. Most of them had been born to poverty-stricken parents at a time when contraception was illegal and when every woman known to be pregnant was subjected to frequent checks to ensure that she had not resorted to illegal abortion. Abandoned and placed in orphanages, the children fell sick through shortages of food and, when hospitalized, received micro-transfusions of untested blood or multiple injections of antibiotics and vitamins using needles and syringes that had probably not been sterilized between uses. In the USSR, investigations of an oubreak involving a chain of hospitals in Kalmykia showed that transmission had begun with the blood from a single HIV-infected child, which had been transferred to uninfected children hospitalized at the same time through a common, shared syringe. Contaminated blood from these newly infected children was in turn transferred, again through improperly sterilized syringes, to yet other children. In all, several hundred children became infected.

Today in eastern Europe and central Asia, HIV is spread mainly through sexual intercourse and, in some countries, through needle-sharing among drug users.

Sexual transmission is the dominant mode of transmission in almost all countries. For example, it accounts for about 80% of the AIDS cases in Bulgaria, the former Czechoslovakia and Hungary. As of 1991, more than 6 in 10 HIV infections reported by Czechoslovakia were in homosexual men, whereas heterosexual transmission predominated in Bulgaria.

HIV infection among injecting drug users is also increasing. Some 57% of AIDS cases in the former Yugoslavia, and 40% in Poland, have been linked to this route. In Poland, studies of drug injectors since 1989 have turned up HIV prevalence rates of 10% or more. Little is known about the extent of HIV/AIDS in people who inject drugs in other countries of the region, although anecdotal evidence suggests that drug injecting is increasing along with social and economic hardship.

While the region is fortunate in still having low levels of HIV infection and AIDS, the situation is volatile. Economic crisis, ethnic and religious conflicts, displacement of civilian populations and disruption of families hinder the ability of the region's health services to offer effective AIDS prevention. These developments also encourage the kinds of behaviour through which HIV can spread. Large-scale rape by soldiers has been reported in some places. Drug use is on the rise, and men and women are in-

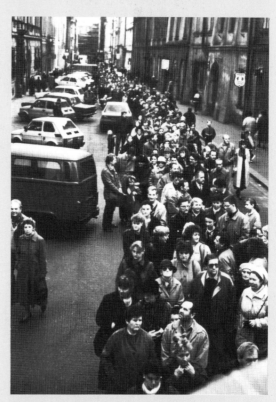

Economic crises, war, displacement of civilian populations and the disruption of families have created ideal conditions for HIV spread in central and eastern Europe. Drug use is on the rise, and women and men are increasingly turning to prostitution. At the same time, information about AIDS is often limited, as are condom supplies.

creasingly turning to prostitution in settings that lack the tradition of community organization which helped prostitutes in western European countries to protect themselves from infection. Even welcome changes such as the freedom to travel, increased tourism and the liberalization of cultural mores may spur transmission.

It is now increasingly recognized that if the region is to use its window of opportunity, it will need to focus on true prevention programmes rather than on the mass HIV testing that has so far absorbed the lion's share of the AIDS budget.

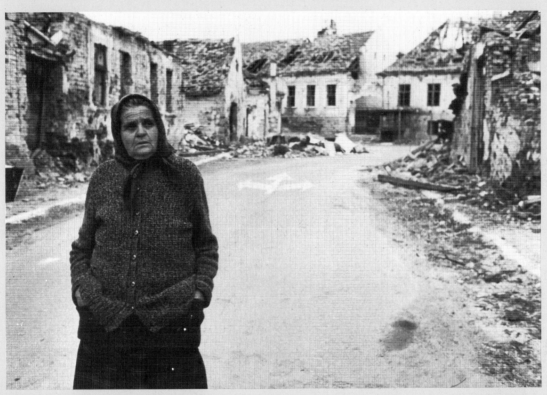

War in the Balkans. Little can be done to stop the spread of HIV in situations where the social infrastructure has been destroyed and communities have been scattered by fighting.

CHAPTER 12

The ripple effect of AIDS

"This part of Kagera close to the lake was always considered blessed; no one had to sweat to feed himself here. Bananas grew all around, there were fish in the lake, and a good climate. Then AIDS came and the blessed life ended." — Odelia Rwenyagira, United Republic of Tanzania (11)

Tum's mother was young, single and HIV-positive. When she went to the maternity hospital to give birth, she checked in under a false name and address and slipped out of the hospital when her baby was only a few hours old. Today the little boy is nearly a year old; with his big eyes and delicate features he is immensely appealing. But until now, no one has offered him a home or family.

HIV-infected women who abandon their babies are often already sick themselves and face an early death. Few can bear the thought of watching their children struggle through a short life should they have passed on the virus during pregnancy.

Though the overwhelming majority of infected mothers do not abandon their offspring, such babies are an increasingly common feature of the AIDS epidemic almost everywhere. But they are part of a far larger phenomenon that is turning out to be one of the most serious social consequences of the epidemic — the phenomenon of AIDS orphans. WHO predicts that by the end of this decade, the mothers of some 5 – 10 million children under 10 years of age worldwide will have died in the epidemic, leaving their offspring to survive alone or in the care of relatives or friends who are often ill-equipped to take on the tough task of raising someone else's children.

AIDS orphans, like the abandoned babies, present a poignant illustration of the far-reaching effects of the epidemic. In this chapter we will explore how this disease, like a stone dropped into a pool, sends out ripples to the very edge of society, affecting first the family, then the community, and then the nation.

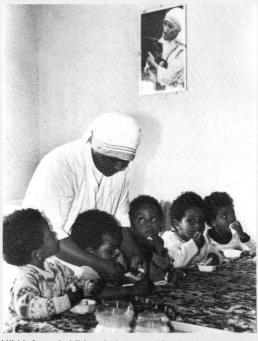

HIV-infected children being cared for in a home in Addis Ababa run by nuns of Mother Teresa's order. No matter how ill, seropositive children can still get a great deal from life—from a kiss, a smile, a sweet, the warm rays of the sun. And they have a lot to give, too, to those who care for them.

Africa's motherless children

The vast majority of the children orphaned by AIDS up to the end of this century will be in sub-Saharan Africa, where formerly the extended family could always be relied upon to take in the dependants of those who died. But today the continent's age-old, traditional social security system — which has proved itself resilient to so many social changes — is buckling under the unprecedented strain of AIDS.

In the Kagera region of the United Republic of Tanzania, the closest and most senior male relative would automatically assume responsibility for the wife and children of a man who died. Today, there are simply too many stranded dependants for any system to cope with. The traditional family has almost totally disappeared in the region, which has been hit simultaneously with blight and pests sweeping

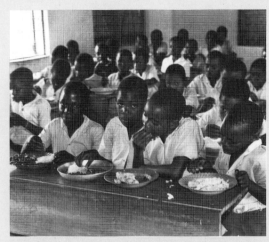

A midday meal for every child in this school is part of a programme to help AIDS orphans. More than 1 in 10 pupils at the school has lost a parent to AIDS, but they are not the only needy children in this poor community — so everyone is fed.

through the banana plantations, decimating the staple food crop.

No one knows exactly how many children are involved, but it is estimated that in east and central Africa alone, between 3.1 and 5.5 million children — that is, 5 – 10% of all children under 15 — will lose their mothers to AIDS during the 1990s. In these countries there are already many households composed of the young and the old left to fend for themselves after the death of the breadwinners.

"In the developing world, social security means not a government check, but having enough able-bodied people in your family to rely on for food and shelter," Dr Michael Merson, Director of WHO's Global Programme on AIDS, told the US Congress in 1992. "AIDS is cutting vast holes in this ancient safety net, and millions of people are falling through. Besides the children who are orphaned, there are huge numbers of elderly people who, having lost their adult children to AIDS, live out their last few years impoverished and alone."

The Odetas from Kagera are an example of a family struggling to survive after the death of all its young adults. Today, six children live with their grandfather, who often drinks to excess, and their grandmother who, since the death of her only son, Dominic, in 1988, has been broken-hearted and ill. They live at the end of a narrow track through tall trees in a house whose cracked walls let in wind, rain and broken shafts of sunlight. But there is no money coming into the house for repairs,

or even for new clothes. Nor is anyone big enough or strong enough to farm the small *shamba*. The family depends on charity and the goodwill of neighbours for everything from labour and food, to school uniforms for the youngsters.

Their mother, who died in 1991, knew how hard life would be for the old folk and the children when she died, and she fought the effects of AIDS as long and hard as she could. Working ceaselessly, she dug and weeded the *shamba*, and started to build a sturdier house for the family. But her strength ebbed before she could finish the house, and today she lies beside its roofless walls in a grave next to her husband's, marked with a wooden cross.

Johannsen Johanna is headmaster of the nearby primary school where more than one in ten of his pupils has lost a parent in the epidemic. Most of the orphans, he says, cannot afford their fees; they come to school without pencils and exercise books, too. But unlike other headmasters who refuse to take children who cannot pay the fees, Mr Johanna cannot turn away his orphans. Their shame at being different from the others as they sit at their desks without equipment or decent uniforms is obvious to see, and frequently their ability to learn is blocked by emotional problems.

"Kids come to school without eating sometimes," said Prudencia Rweyemera, one of the teachers. "They fall asleep on their desks,

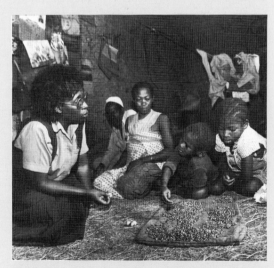

Odelia Rwenyagira of the Rubya home-based care team visits the Odeta family. Since the death of their parents, the six children live with their grandmother and grandfather in a dilapidated house. But with all the family's breadwinners gone, there is no money for house repairs, new clothes, or even schooling for some of the kids.

and I have to take them back to my home to give them a meal.''

Many who cannot take the hardship and humiliation simply drop out of school, and some end up very young, unskilled and full of frustration on the streets of nearby towns. ''Places like Mwanza and Bukoba [on the shores of Lake Victoria] never had problems with street children before,'' said a nurse-educator working in Kagera. ''But now there are little gangs of orphaned kids who have run away from their villages and who live by robbing people.''

With no family or school life to socialize these children or develop their potential, they may never be able to play a constructive role in society. ''AIDS orphans will undoubtedly pose one of the greatest challenges to economic development in Africa in recent history,'' says Elizabeth Preble, former AIDS advisor for UNICEF (*12*).

The crippling cost of illness

By the time parents die, their children and elderly dependants are often deeply impoverished because of the costs in time and money of caring for someone with AIDS. In Zaire, a single admission to Kinshasa's main hospital, Mama Yemo, for a child with AIDS costs the equivalent of several months of an average salary, and funerals cost the equivalent of nearly one year's salary. And in Thailand, lifetime health care costs per person with AIDS are estimated at a minimum of US$1000, which is 30–50% of the annual income of the average Thai family (*13*).

The struggle at family level to shoulder the burden of AIDS is mirrored at the national level. In the United Republic of Tanzania the national health budget is US$5 per head — less than the cost of a single blood test for HIV.

Spelling out the crisis facing the health services in Ethiopia in 1992, Dr Bona Hora, at that time head of the AIDS programme, said: ''We have a total of 11 000 hospital beds, and by the end of this year we are expecting to have nearly 26 000 adult cases of AIDS, and perhaps 12 000 paediatric cases.'' In many of the large hospitals of Central and East Africa, 20–40% of beds are already occupied by peo-

ple with AIDS, and rates in some others are higher still.

In developed countries too, the epidemic is making significant demands on health services, and these demands will increase as people already infected with HIV develop AIDS. The cost of caring for an AIDS patient from diagnosis to death in the USA, for instance, has been calculated at $50 000 – $60 000 (*14*), and by 1991 such patients were expected to account for twice as many hospital bed–days per year as lung cancer — one of the nation's leading causes of death.

It has been estimated that in 1992 the cost of medical care for some half a million people with AIDS was close to US$ 5000 million. Industrialized countries accounted for over 90% of these costs although they accounted for only 22% of the cases. But almost 80% of the world's new infections are now occurring in the developing world. The burden on these nations — including some of the poorest countries in the world — can only grow. In the remaining years of this decade, the developing countries will spend over US$ 1000 million on health care for AIDS patients.

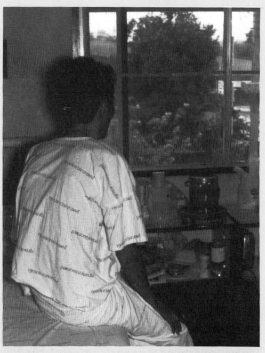

A man with AIDS in a Bangkok hospital. In Thailand the cost of treating one patient with AIDS is far greater than what the government budgets for all health care per person.

The impact of AIDS deaths

Using special modelling techniques, WHO and the World Bank have provided a picture of the likely demographic impact of AIDS deaths on a hypothetical sub-Saharan country with a current high prevalence of HIV. Between 1985 and 1990 in this country, the death rate rose by 0.3 per 1000 population as a result of AIDS deaths, and a further increase of 1.1 per 1000 population is expected by the mid-1990s. In the absence of AIDS, death rates would have been expected to start declining from 1985.

Because so many factors that might affect the picture are unknown or unpredictable, there are inherent limitations in such projections. However, the model indicates the following:

- Life expectancy for a person born in this hypothetical country will decrease from about 50 years in 1985 to 47 in the year 2010. In the absence of AIDS, life expectancy would have grown by more than 11 years.
- Between 1985 and 1990, AIDS added an average of 10% to the annual death rate for people aged 15 – 49; by the mid-1990s, it will increase adult death rates by more than 40%. These projections are for the country as a whole: in the worst-affected urban areas, adult deaths are expected to double or triple.
- By the mid-1990s, infant mortality is expected to be 4% higher than it would be in the absence of AIDS. By this time, too, AIDS deaths in children will begin to reverse the progress made over the past two decades in child survival through programmes such as immunization and oral rehydration of children with diarrhoea.
- The heavy toll of deaths in children under 5 and those aged 15 – 44 is not expected to result in an actual decline in the size of the population in this hypothetical country, nor in any sub-Saharan African country. It will merely slow down the population's growth rate. The population — which grew by about 3.4% in 1990 — would be growing by 2.4% a year by 2010, instead of by around 3%, as it would in the absence of AIDS.

Thus the most dramatic demographic impact will be not on the size of the population, but on its age structure. As young and middle-aged adults are picked off by AIDS, there will be disproportionate numbers of old

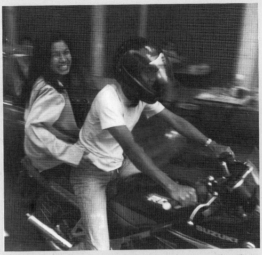

Young couple, Thailand. AIDS disproportionately affects young adults who are in the prime of their working years. In many countries, the loss to the economy stemming from the loss of their productivity will be far greater than the cost of their health care.

people and, especially, children in the population, skewing the "population age pyramid".

It is this that ensures that the economic effects of the epidemic will be felt far beyond the health sector, for countries will lose their most productive members, the men and women on whom the economy depends. In many countries, their loss will undermine the development process itself.

There have been relatively few detailed studies of overall economic impact in developing countries, but some data from Thailand are instructive. These show that the direct health care costs of AIDS — around $1000 a year per patient — are dwarfed by the indirect costs of the premature illness and death of adults in the prime of their working years, which the Thai economists estimate at $22 000 per death (equal to approximately 14 times the 1991 gross national product per capita).

Their study also concludes that, in aggregate, these costs are enormous. Health care costs plus the value of lost income and other indirect costs to the nation will rise from $100 million in 1991 to a maximum of $2200 million by the year 2000 (or a minimum of $1800 million, in the best-case scenario). Looked at another way, during the 1990s, between $7300 million and $8700 million will have been lost to the Thai economy as a result of AIDS illness and death (15).

Giving an indication of the economic impact in Africa, WHO has calculated that AIDS

AIDS-impoverished families

There are endless stories of families selling their possessions and even the land on their doorsteps in desperate bids for treatment or a cure.

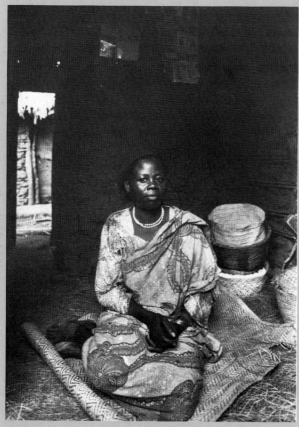

Feliciana Josephat and her children were left impoverished by her late husband's long illness and his frantic and costly search for an AIDS cure.

Feliciana Josephat's husband refused for months to believe that he had AIDS; certain that he had been bewitched, he spent all the family's savings on futile visits to the witch doctor. When he finally recognized the nature of his illness he sold off bits of his *shamba* to buy medicines on the black market. He died in 1988 leaving his six children and his wife, who was already suffering from AIDS herself, with nothing. Sometimes the children are turned away from school because they cannot pay the small fee. When Feliciana is fit enough, she labours on other people's farms; and when she is too ill to work the family simply goes without food. Already they rise and retire with the sun, for Feliciana cannot afford even candles to light the tiny house after dark.

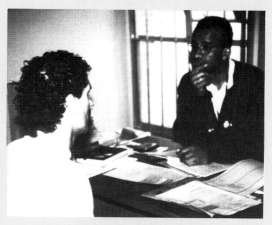

A counselling session at the AIDS Reference and Training Center, São Paulo, Brazil. Almost 80% of the world's new HIV infections are occurring in the developing world.

deaths in Uganda will triple the number of potentially productive years lost in the 20–50 age group. And researchers at Harvard University predicted that economic losses as a result of AIDS in five badly affected central African countries would exceed the total inflow of foreign aid to those countries by 1991.

The economic impact on industrialized countries will also be substantial but it will not be overwhelming simply because these countries are rich. The developing countries will be hit immeasurably harder both because their baseline economies are so much weaker *and* because they will be shouldering 90% of the world's HIV infections by the year 2000.

It is easier to predict the explosive impact of the AIDS epidemic than to foresee how the pieces will fall. Societies and economies are dynamic, and the good news from past epidemics is that people and institutions are flexible and can accommodate considerable change. However, societies will be unable to make the most of their potential flexibility unless they take the epidemic seriously and start now to analyse, sector by sector, what AIDS will mean for the economy.

As a special panel set up by the US National Research Council stresses, ''Difficult though it might be to predict the future import of the present impact of the HIV/AIDS epidemic, one should not shrink from the task, especially when one must plan for the future'' (*16*).

PART III

Why is AIDS still spreading?

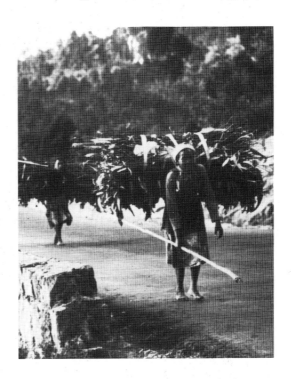

CHAPTER 13

An opportunistic virus

"HIV feeds on our weaknesses. It thrives on our cultural reluctance to discuss sexuality. It exploits our ancient societal weaknesses... [and] plays on our spiritual weaknesses, especially fear and intolerance." — Dr Michael H. Merson, Director, WHO Global Programme on AIDS (17)

The worldwide fight against AIDS has seen an unprecedented mobilization of forces and many achievements. National AIDS programmes have been set up with the help of the World Health Organization in practically every developing country. There has been intense activity at grassroots level as hundreds of specialist AIDS service organizations have come into being, and existing nongovernmental organizations working in community development have taken on the challenge of AIDS.

However, the campaign is up against formidable obstacles. AIDS follows the ancient fault-lines in society, taking advantage of some of humanity's most intractable problems such as poverty and discrimination. HIV is an "opportunistic" virus in the sense that it exploits ignorance, prejudice, fear, fatalism — and the very human tendency to hide from difficult or threatening truths in the hope that they will go away of their own accord.

"AIDS won't affect us"

"A lesson from earlier epidemics is the danger of complacency, even denial that a catastrophe is in the making," Dr Michael Merson, Director of WHO's Global Programme on AIDS, told delegates to a Latin American AIDS conference in 1991. "Complacency about HIV infection is especially dangerous because infection is invisible for so long." By the time people die off in great numbers, the virus has spread deep into the community.

Yet in practically every country that now has a national AIDS campaign, governments initially lost valuable time before admitting they were affected by a disease that carries a devastating social stigma. Many countries were understandably worried about the possible effects on tourism and investment; and some were — and often still are — simply too preoccupied by war,

natural disasters or economic problems to take on yet another catastrophe.

Some countries maintain that their cultural and moral traditions ensure that they will never get a disease they associate with deviance. A major stumbling block is the association of AIDS with homosexuality — a behaviour so taboo in many cultures that, rather than acknowledge it, people would prefer to believe it does not exist among them, or only on the fringes of society where people may have been influenced by contact with "decadent" foreign cultures.

In some countries this line of argument is extended to other forms of behaviour consi-

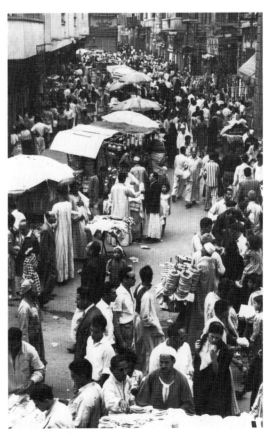

No country has been immune to HIV, and none will remain unaffected by AIDS. The behaviours through which HIV is transmitted occur to a greater or lesser extent in all societies.

dered deviant, such as sex with multiple partners, prostitution and drug-taking. The rationale for inaction is the belief that any outbreak of HIV infection will remain within marginalized groups and never pose a threat to the wider population. Experience shows, however, that this does not happen: *nowhere has the virus remained confined to any specific population group.*

Denial has been part of the response to AIDS in virtually every country. For example, a government official in India said, in 1991: "Considering our social and cultural values and traditions, I feel quite confident that AIDS will not spread as far and fast as in Africa." In 1990 an official of the then Soviet Union said: "The roots of [HIV] spread are the American and Western way of life, unrestrained and flourishing homosexuality, drugs and obsession with sex." It is telling that views in both these parts of the world have changed since.

Risk behaviour is universal

Sexual behaviour that is risky in the context of AIDS — unprotected intercourse with multiple partners — is universal.

Sex between males occurs in every society and has been observed among other primates too. But where there is no social acceptance of male homosexuality, AIDS prevention programmes run into a serious obstacle: secrecy. "In many countries getting married and having children are not so much matters of choice as of social survival, and there is little scope to deviate from this norm," explains Meurig Horton of GPA's high-risk behaviour unit. "It follows that, in such places, many men who are homosexual by preference will be family men whose relationships with other men have to be kept secret."

Surveys in Africa, where homosexuality is strictly taboo and widely denied, found that 15% of male respondents in Botswana acknowledged having had homosexual encounters; 18.6% of 586 people interviewed in eastern Uganda said they knew about bisexuality and 16% reported having had sex with both men and women; and in Egypt 10% of men interviewed at a clinic for sexually transmitted diseases claimed to be bisexual and another 9% homosexual (*18*). "Men do have sex with each

other, but it's not called homosexuality. It doesn't have a name; it's just something that's done," said a gay man from Sierra Leone. "In most of Africa it's like that" (*19*).

Social scientists investigating the world of female sex workers in Ethiopia were taken by surprise when the focus groups ventured, unsolicited, the information that young men — many of them students needing money to finance their studies — are selling sex in ever-increasing numbers on the streets of Addis Ababa. And in countries of central and eastern Europe where homosexuals, for decades, had to hide their sexual identity because of social and political repression, the past few years have seen the first stirrings of "gay liberation" as people have begun to come out of the closet and to organize on their own behalf.

As far as heterosexual risk behaviour is concerned, the records of family planning clinics, STD clinics and maternity hospitals bear witness to the fact that sexual activity outside marriage goes on in even the most conservative societies. Indeed, some bizarre stratagems are used to make the act of sex with casual partners fit the prevailing ethos. In a few places in the Islamic world, for example, the custom of taking "temporary wives" has been adopted, which allows a man to "marry" for sex and divorce immediately afterwards. Thus sexual intercourse takes place within a context that is sanctioned by law, religion and culture.

Another form of denial is to acknowledge the behaviour, but not the risk it carries. For example, in societies where heterosexual intercourse outside marriage is recognized as common, as in the USA and Europe, some people continue to assert that this is not how HIV is spread in *their* countries and accuse experts who say otherwise of deliberately deceiving the public. The fact that heterosexual spread in these countries has not been as explosive as some predicted is taken irrationally as justification for this position, rather than as an indication of the great difficulty of forecasting the path of such a virus.

Unless countries acknowledge the full diversity of behaviour practised within their borders, and its implications for the spread of HIV, the containment of AIDS is impossible. Effective education and behaviour change depend on frank and open discussion about HIV transmission and the measures people can take to protect themselves.

The power of ignorance

Although many millions of dollars have been spent worldwide on information and education, the messages are hard to get through. Many people continue to deny that AIDS has any relevance to their own lives. Myths and misconceptions abound.

As late as 1990, in the USA, the world's largest information telephone service, the National AIDS Hotline, was receiving 3000 calls a day from people wondering if they could catch AIDS through handshakes, toilet seats or popcorn served by someone with HIV. In parts of Africa, men, knowing AIDS is associated with wasting, believe sex with a plump woman is "safe". Others are convinced that an HIV-infected man can rid himself of the virus through sex with a virgin.

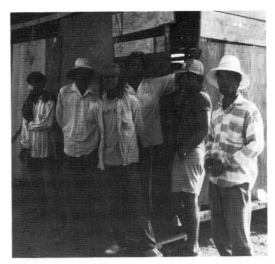

Denial of the AIDS threat takes many forms. These construction workers on a building site near Bangkok expressed the opinion that AIDS was just a myth created by condom manufacturers to induce people to buy their product.

A battle with intolerance

"In the black community the concept of homosexuality had never really been discussed until recently," said Simon Nkoli of the Township AIDS Project in Soweto, South Africa. "It's still a taboo; we find a lot of black people who are anti-gay, and sometimes if people find out you're gay, you get physically assaulted."

Nkoli is a leading member of the Gay and Lesbian Organization of the Witwatersrand (GLOW), a multiracial organization founded in 1988 to fight for gay rights as part of South Africa's wider liberation struggle, and to inform gay people about issues concerning them, such as AIDS. "The problem in the black community is the very slow pace of getting proper information. Things are written, but there are lots of people who are illiterate," said Nkoli.

"To the black community, admitting you're gay is to be immediately labelled 'an AIDS carrier'. Or, if someone is found to have the disease, people may say: 'But I thought he is married. Maybe he went to prison and got it there?' There's a lot of ignorance because of poor education. In the past few years when we talked about AIDS, people were laughing at us — even gay men were laughing — because they didn't think it was anything to do with them. GLOW had a big campaign against AIDS. We were holding talks in all our chapters, and black people were saying: 'Forget it, I'm not a white man and I don't have a white lover'. People also believed that because they didn't come from central Africa they wouldn't get it.

"But now we have workshops and it's so exciting to see how things have changed. Gay black men are concerned about being careful. But resources are a real problem. We talked about condoms, but where could we get them? They're so expensive. The chemist's price is R15 [approximately US$ 6] for twelve condoms, and people don't have that kind of money. Some went to family planning clinics, but they wouldn't give condoms to gays."

The battle for respect, human rights, and the means of protection from HIV is an uphill struggle. South Africa was the scene, in 1990, of the first Gay Liberation March on the African continent, when around 800 gay people created a carnival atmosphere with their banners, costumes and music in the streets of Johannesburg. But it is also the place where British Sgxabai, a very popular gay rights campaigner and member of GLOW, was savagely beaten with a garden fork by one of his family when he returned home with teeshirts and condoms after an AIDS workshop. He died soon after in hospital.

"Sgxabai will be for us what Steve Biko [a black anti-apartheid activist who died in police detention] was for all black people — a tragic symbol of our oppression," said his friend Simon Nkoli.

To an extent these fantasies are the result of a proliferation of complex and often contradictory information. For example, pictures of police wearing protective clothing when dealing with people they think might have HIV contradict the message that casual contact is not a threat.

Sometimes messages are rejected because they conflict with cultural assumptions. "They say it's a virus that's made me sick, but I know it's witchcraft," said a patient in an African AIDS hospice, intimating that he humoured the nurses for the sake of peace.

Sometimes ignorance is the result of misinformation. And sometimes it is a question of people having little faith in the source of the information or the "messenger" bringing it. "The media shove some figures down your throat. They've made it worse than it really is so they can stop you having sex," said a teenage boy in Norfolk, England (20). In parts of Africa, blacks look on AIDS information provided through official government channels as a ploy by whites to curtail black sexual activity and slow down black population growth. And in Thailand, construction workers commented that all the talk about AIDS is a marketing trick by condom manufacturers.

The fact that many people have never seen anyone with AIDS denies them a basis for believing that AIDS exists, and people with AIDS (PWA) who are prepared to reveal their status therefore play a vital role in awakening their communities to the reality of the epidemic. "So much can be done when people with AIDS are used as educators," says Donald de Gagné, a director of the Vancouver PWA Society. "Young kids will listen attentively to a person with AIDS and be marked by the experience. That is much more effective than a public health person talking about AIDS in the abstract. But we do not have a place in the sun yet. It is still very hard to get people to come out and be visible when they will face human rights abuses."

Ignorance or rejection of the facts is a

Blighted lives

Tales of stigma and persecution come from all corners of the world:

• "We have to protect the records of people who test positive for HIV as carefully as any official secret because of the public attitude," commented Dr Supachai Rerks-ngarm, Director of the AIDS Division, Ministry of Public Health, who said that suicide occurs in Thailand among people with HIV. Regrettably, said Dr Supachai, discrimination against HIV-infected people appears to have been encouraged by Thailand's early education and information campaigns. "We set out to scare people about the disease, but I think we made them scared about people with the disease instead. We learnt a lot from that and our education campaign now aims to encourage compassion in the public."

• "There were no support groups, no social workers, nobody, so I retreated further into my community," said Willie Bettelyoun of the USA. "But even that was wrong. I had people coming to my door wanting to beat me up — they didn't want AIDS in their community — even though these were my relatives. Because I had AIDS I was no longer human. I was a disease. I no longer had feelings. I no longer was given the opportunity to plan, to have goals, to contribute" (3).

• "A friend of mine — a man of 22 who was a health worker — kept being admitted to hospital for malaria," a young man told a gathering of medical people in southern Africa. "One day when I went to visit, I found him not in the usual ward but alone in a side room with a sticker on the door saying 'isolated'. There was a bucket to use as a toilet because he was not allowed out of the room. I found him shocked: he had no idea what was going on. A nurse told me the staff had been ordered by matron not to go into the room. That evening the consultant told my friend that he had AIDS and he had not got long to live. My friend had never heard anything at all about AIDS and he became kind of hysterical at the news" (21).

• In London, according to a spokesman for BHAN (the Black HIV and AIDS Network), there are examples of people with HIV infection or AIDS travelling to the far side of the city to see a doctor or social worker rather than risk bumping into someone they know at the local hospital. This is particularly common among marginalized minorities — people whose communities are often a refuge from a hostile environment, and for whom losing acceptance would cause deep misery.

powerful barrier to the containment of AIDS. If people believe — wrongly — that they can be infected with HIV through casual contact or mosquitos, they may see little point in modifying their sexual or drug-injecting behaviour.

Ignorance also gives free rein to fear, prejudice, and the impulse to discriminate. These reactions are so widespread that a human rights organization comments: "People with HIV/AIDS face double jeopardy. They face death, and while they are fighting for their lives, they often face discrimination. This is manifested in all areas of life — from health care to housing, from education to work to travel. Whereas most illnesses produce sympathy and support from family, friends and neighbours, persons with AIDS are frequently feared and shunned" (*22*).

So strong is the stigma that even seropositive people sometimes subscribe to prejudices they have internalized. "The first time I went to a meeting of a support group for HIV-positive people," said a young Brazilian living in Paris, "I was really surprised to see the six people in the group, including a man in his 60s and two women. What struck me was that these were just 'ordinary people'. It took me a long time to get the courage to go to the group, and I think I had expected to see freaks of some kind."

The false lure of isolation

In an atmosphere of public prejudice and hysteria, many governments' first response is to try to identify and isolate those with the virus. A number of countries insist on foreign workers, students or potential immigrants being tested for HIV, and deny entry to those who test positive. Prisons and hospitals often segregate people with the virus. And there are numerous examples of people being tested compulsorily and then detained in prisons, camps or hospitals if found to be infected.

In Cuba this "test and isolate" approach has been taken to its logical conclusion. People identified as HIV-positive through a programme of compulsory testing have been sent to special AIDS sanatoria, sometimes called "sidatoria". Inmates have been allowed to visit their families on occasional weekends, or to leave the sanatorium for business purposes, with

> The history of epidemics shows that the instinct to blame and to isolate those believed to be responsible is a common response. Isolation of those affected by past epidemics such as smallpox, plague and tuberculosis may be understandable — because these diseases are contagious through everyday contact — although quarantine has never been an unqualified success. But in the case of AIDS, which is not "contagious", isolation is not only a gross human rights violation: it is pointless and even dangerous.

a "chaperone", if deemed necessary by the authorities.

But mandatory isolation has failed to stop the spread of the virus in Cuba — additional sanatoria have had to be opened. The only way to contain HIV is to help people adopt safer behaviour. Recognizing this, Cuban authorities announced at the World Health Assembly in May 1993 that as from June isolation would no longer be mandatory. Infected people are to be given the choice between living in the sanatorium and living at home and receiving care as an outpatient.

Attempts to isolate or publicly identify people with HIV/AIDS are thus pointless. What is worse, they can actually fuel the spread of HIV. For one thing, they breed complacency in others. The people outside the stigmatized, "tested" group feel invulnerable, and then fail to make necessary changes in their behaviour, even though there is no way to identify everyone who is carrying the virus.

The effects of stimulating a false sense of security are well illustrated in Germany where, in certain towns, prostitutes are required to be checked for certain STDs every week and are given health inspection cards. Many customers think these cards "guarantee" against disease and so refuse to use condoms.

The problem is not confined to Germany. A European shipbroker whose work frequently takes him to south-east Asia, where he has a regular sex partner, said: "I tell her when I'm due to arrive and she has an HIV test just before. If she has an up-to-date health card I know I'm safe."

In fact, a negative HIV test is no guarantee that a person is not infected. Fabricated test cards can be bought in many countries. At best, a test result is no more than a momentary snapshot of somebody's status. The person may become infected in the days or even hours following the test, or may already be infected but still in the "window period" of infection (i.e. the period before antibodies to the virus are detectable in the blood). And how often can the costly and time-consuming exercise of HIV testing be carried out?

Since customers are not forced or even expected to disclose their health status, a rule such as this, which gives clients an excuse not to use condoms, only increases the sex workers' vulnerability to HIV infection.

There are further problems. Besides stimulating a false sense of security in the not-yet-infected, discrimination encourages secrecy in those who *are* infected, or think they might be. It makes them afraid of contact with the health and social services they so badly need. And by driving underground those with personal experience of HIV/AIDS, it silences people who would otherwise be the epidemic's most credible and sensitive witnesses, and invaluable allies in the fight against AIDS.

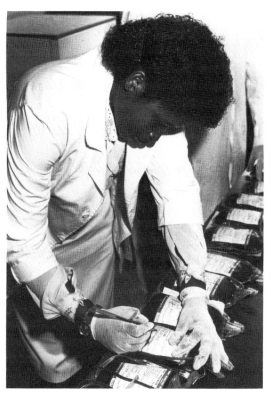

Mandatory HIV testing makes sense only for keeping the blood supply safe.

CHAPTER 14

AIDS and poverty: a deadly symbiosis

"Poverty makes whole communities vulnerable to AIDS by forcing men to leave their families in search of work, by leaving people hopeless enough to turn to the solace of drugs, or by making prostitution a survival strategy for women and children. AIDS then completes the vicious circle by making the community even poorer" (23).

A look at a map of the world shaded according to HIV prevalence tells a story that cannot be ignored, for much of the heavy shading — indicating the areas on which the epidemic has its tightest grip — covers the poorest countries. And the highest concentrations of HIV/AIDS within *rich* countries coincide increasingly with pockets of misery and deprivation, mostly in urban slums.

This underlines a truth that is fundamental to the understanding of the epidemic — that poverty is at once the line of least resistance, and one of the most powerful driving forces behind the spread of AIDS. It eases the path of the virus through a variety of complex and overlapping mechanisms.

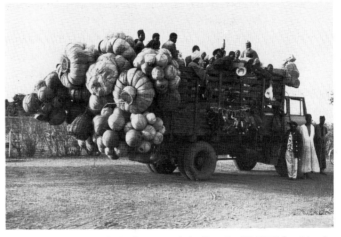

Migration, often the result of poverty, is fuelling the HIV/AIDS epidemic. Male migrants are drawn to the cities, creating a male-female imbalance in the urban population that makes casual (and particularly commercial) sex more likely. In cities such as Harare and Nairobi, men outnumber women by as much as 3 to 2.

Far from home

The decision to leave home involves both elements of "need to leave" and "desire to be elsewhere". The economic boom in parts of Asia, for example, has drawn people from far and wide with the promise of jobs in new industries. But if opportunities and the prospect of adventure and bright city lights are the "pull" factors, poverty is overwhelmingly the "push" factor. Throughout the world, the struggle to survive in depressed or underdeveloped areas drives people to try their luck elsewhere. This has always been so. What is new is the scale of it: today, unprecedented numbers of people are on the move from countryside to city, from city to city, and from country to country in pursuit of work that will lift themselves and their families off the treadmill of need.

It is a migration that often takes the heart out of communities, disrupting family life and stable relationships and loosening traditional controls on behaviour. Men and women try to reconstruct their lives far from home, taking new sex partners during their long absences. Furthermore, many who leave their homes in search of work find that prostitution offers the best, and sometimes the only, way of earning a living.

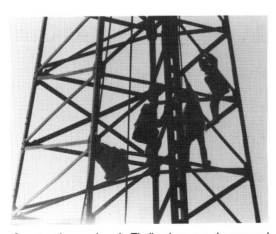

Construction workers in Thailand are mostly seasonal migrants from poor rural areas who spend months each year away from home. Their unsettled lifestyle makes them particularly vulnerable to HIV, and they account for a large proportion of the country's AIDS cases to date.

The link between poverty-driven migration and AIDS is clearly demonstrated in Thailand. According to Jon Ungphakorn, director of the Bangkok organization ACCESS, the roots of the present AIDS crisis in his country can be traced to "national development policies over the past three decades which have focused on rapid overall economic growth at the expense of all other considerations" (9).

In the single-minded pursuit of industrialization, investment in the rural areas has been neglected and traditionally self-reliant farming communities have sunk into poverty and debt, forcing people to migrate in search of work. As of mid-1991, the occupational groups worst affected by HIV in Thailand were male construction workers, fishermen and female sex workers, many of whom are recent immigrants from rural areas.

Children caught in the trap

Children, too, are being pushed out of their homes by poverty and into situations where they are at increased risk of contracting HIV. Throughout the world more than 100 mil-

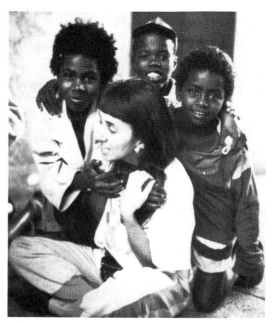

Street kids in Brazil. Worldwide, 100 million kids are living rough on the streets. Risk-taking is a daily part of life on the margin of society, and such children are vulnerable to HIV infection from sexual or drug-taking behaviour. Few know the facts about HIV.

lion kids live rough on the streets, abandoned by parents who cannot afford to feed and clothe them, or having run away from conditions they found intolerable. Around 20 million of these children are on the streets of the industrialized world, 40 million in Latin America, 30 million in Asia and 10 million in Africa.

Street children are extremely vulnerable to HIV infection, both because they are outside all formal structures of society such as school, and hence are difficult to reach with health education and health care; and because risk-taking is part and parcel of existence on the knife-edge of survival. Many use drugs to escape from their pain — a habit that ranges from sniffing glue to injecting heroin or cocaine.

However, hard drugs are usually way beyond the means of destitute children, and their biggest risk of contracting HIV comes from sex. Many have run away from sexual abuse at home, only to face more abuse from older boys and adults on the streets. Some are at risk of HIV infection through sexual relationships they form with other youngsters on the streets, who are often their only source of physical and emotional comfort. And some sell sex to survive: homeless kids living by prostitution are a feature of cities and busy ports from South America to south-east Asia, Africa, Europe and the USA.

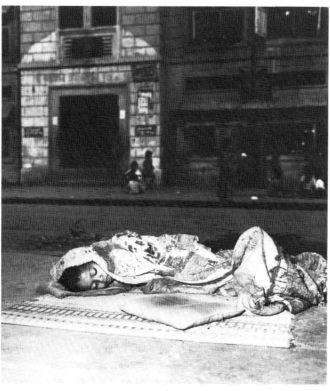

The pavement is home to this Asian child.

In the Philippines 50 000–75 000 street children are believed to live by prostitution (24).

But juvenile prostitution is not limited to survival on the streets. Sometimes poor parents sell their children to middle men who come to the villages in search of labour — usually with some awareness that "hotel jobs" are in fact prostitution. The dynamics behind this commerce in northern Thailand have already been described in Chapter 6. But the same phenomenon exists in other countries where opportunities for making a living are few and far between, and where there are people ready to exploit the children of poor families.

For example, certain Asian countries have, for the past 20 years or so, been destinations for men, mostly European, seeking sex with boys. Over recent years the trade has become more organized. Said an AIDS expert who recently visited the region: "Today a tourist can rent the services of a boy at the same time as he rents his accommodation and books his flight. Tour operators based in Europe are offering such package deals."

"High-risk environments"

Poverty not only imposes on people patterns of living which increase their risk of exposure to HIV, but it often robs them of the knowledge or the means to protect themselves.

AIDS information campaigns — together with the research and planning needed to ensure they are effective — are extremely costly. Yet the total budget of national AIDS programmes in some parts of the world is less than the cost of caring for a handful of people with AIDS in the USA. Africa, for instance, is trying to stem the tide of new HIV infections while the continent is sliding further into debt and poverty, per capita gross national product in many countries is lower than it was a decade ago, and many government ministries operate on budgets reduced from year to year. To make matters worse, in many parts of the developing world, educational facilities are poor and illiteracy rates high (especially among women), making it even more difficult to reach large segments of the population with information about AIDS.

Despite the severe handicaps, surveys show that many developing countries have

Wealth and poverty: a paradox

Paradoxically, AIDS in some of the least developed countries is as much a disease of the rich as of the poor. Indeed, in the United Republic of Tanzania, as stated earlier, AIDS was initially dubbed "the disease of money" because the first people affected seemed to be prosperous merchants trading around Lake Victoria.

In Rwanda almost one-third of a sample of people with HIV infection had been through secondary school or higher education, which is suggestive of higher-than-average incomes. And in Zambia one-third of a similar sample had had more than 14 years' schooling (25).

In Malawi a survey of risk factors for HIV infection among 5500 pregnant women, of whom 23% were HIV-positive, found that the women whose husbands or partners were of a high socioeconomic status appeared to be at much greater risk of infection than those whose men were less well-off (25). In Ethiopia, the highest proportions of known AIDS cases have occurred among government officials and former members of the armed forces. During the 1990s, some African countries will lose 10–15% of their middle-class people — the industrial workers, businessmen, teachers, doctors, and politicians on whom they depend for leadership and economic development (26).

The fact is that men with money in their pockets can more easily afford to travel, visit bars and pay for sex than others.

In the developed world, too, many of the early AIDS cases were among the well-to-do and widely travelled. However, these are the people most easily reached and convinced by AIDS information and with readiest access to services, including a supply of condoms.

While well-off people have represented an early wave of infection almost everywhere, it is among the poor in all countries, for whom AIDS prevention is most difficult for all the reasons discussed, that HIV is now spreading fastest.

achieved remarkable successes in informing their populations about AIDS. However, their efforts continue to be undermined by chronic shortages of the basic necessities for HIV prevention such as disposable syringes, test kits for screening blood, rubber gloves, and — most important of all — condoms. Under such circumstances, the concept of "high-risk environments" is at least as important to the analysis as "high-risk behaviour", since people in such environments can do little to protect themselves against HIV infection, no matter how well informed or well intentioned they are.

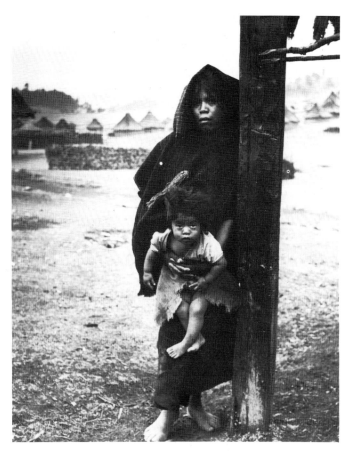

Poverty facilitates risk behaviour and hinders AIDS prevention.

"Shortages of gloves and disposable syringes? We don't even have enough new razor blades to shave the heads of children before setting up a drip," says Dr Lulu Muhe, head of the paediatric section of Addis Ababa's Black Lion Hospital, waving his arm across a ward full of his small patients. Several are already bald, while others wait their turn to be shaved by the nurse kneeling, with a half-shaven child in her arms, in a pile of curly black locks. Dr Muhe's unit is responsible for the care of all known HIV-positive babies and children in Addis Ababa. "I don't think people outside have any conception of the conditions we're working under," he says. "We have to perform lumbar punctures and blood transfusions without gloves. And on top of the shortages there is the workload, which is ever increasing. We get tired and then we get careless."

Shortages affect the treatment of AIDS patients, too. According to staff at the nearby Armed Forces hospital, many of the drugs needed to treat common opportunistic infections are not available, and laboratories lack the necessary equipment, reagents and skills to make effective diagnoses. "For instance," said a doc-

tor, "we often don't know exactly what is causing a patient's diarrhoea." Despite these conditions, committed health staff continue to do all they can to relieve suffering and safeguard human dignity.

Conditions in the hospitals of Ethiopia — where 17 years of civil war have destroyed the economy and the health infrastructure — are by no means unusual: the situation is similar in many poor or war-torn countries. In the United Republic of Tanzania, blood test kits are sometimes out of date when they arrive in the country, or get spoiled by the heat in places where there is no refrigerator available for storage. And in Zaire following widespread riots in late 1991, the supply of test kits to the main blood bank was cut off, and hospitals had to transfuse patients with unscreened blood.

However, since the vast majority of the world's infections are contracted through unprotected intercourse, the most serious poverty-induced shortage is condoms. It is not just a question of money, although this is tremendous — WHO calculates that between US$640 million and US$1160 million per year would be needed to provide adequate supplies of condoms to developing countries — but also of logistics. In many developing countries the infrastructure is rudimentary, and it is harder to ensure regular supplies of all kinds of commodities than when settlements are within reach of good roads and reliable transport systems.

In the hill villages of Kagera bordering Lake Victoria, for example, condoms are available in few of the local shops or kiosks. To help protect people in this area of high mobility and high HIV prevalence, their leaders have instead tried, without much success, to curtail opportunities for sexual encounters by rescheduling weddings and other party occasions to daylight hours.

All manner of problems other than bad roads may block condom distribution. "Sometimes a consignment of condoms is air-freighted to a country at great cost because of urgent need — only to be left standing for months on the tarmac waiting to be cleared through customs," says Dr Patrick Friel, GPA's condom specialist. "Such things are not uncommon." Sometimes corruption and the need to pay bribes to ensure clearance and transportation cause problems. And sometimes the lack of clear lines of responsibility makes distribution erratic. "In some countries there's a long-established tradition of dependency on outside agencies,'' says Friel. ''The attitude is that supplies have always been free; if something goes wrong with a delivery, the donor will send more. It's an attitude that needs to be overcome through proper training of personnel.''

Besides ensuring that condoms are readily available, preventing the sexual spread of HIV means preventing and treating the other STDs that increase people's vulnerability to the virus. This is now seen as an essential part of every effective AIDS programme, yet it too faces many obstacles in poor countries. WHO estimates that effective STD treatment would cost the developing world as a whole up to US$ 1015 million per year.

STD control depends on a properly functioning health system and, in particular, a reliable drug supply, according to Dr Peter Piot, Associate Director of GPA, who is responsible for the area of sexually transmitted diseases within the Programme. ''In countries where there are no drugs or where there is complete chaos, STD control becomes very difficult, if not impossible. Just as you cannot do AIDS prevention without condoms, or needle exchange programmes without needles, you cannot do STD control without drugs.''

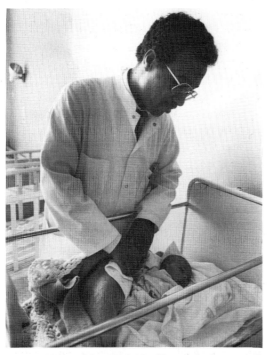

Dr Lulu Muhe of the Black Lion Hospital whose paediatric unit gives care to many HIV-infected children. Here he looks at the newest arrival on his ward — a newborn baby found abandoned on church steps.

A synergy of plagues

In the rich world it is the poorest communities that bear the brunt of HIV infection and disease. In the USA, for example, Hispanics — 25% of whom live below the poverty line, as compared with a national figure of 10% for all ethnic groups combined — constituted 16% of AIDS cases in 1991, but only 9% of the population. African-Americans, whose poverty is even worse, constituted 12% of the population but nearly 28% of AIDS cases. In 1992, AIDS rates in black women were over 30 per 100 000, as compared with less than 2 per 100 000 for white women.

Following an extensive fact-finding mission across the country, the US National Commission on AIDS reported in 1991: ''HIV disease [cannot] be understood outside the context of racism, homophobia, poverty, and unemployment — pervasive factors that foster the spread of the disease. This web of associated social ills has been referred to as 'a synergy of plagues'.

''Poverty and unemployment in the inner-cities of the US entail much more than an inability to pay the bills,'' continued the report. ''In 1991 being poor is a generic risk factor, for it is associated with increased risk of becoming homeless, dying a violent death, and suffering perhaps from a multitude of preventable illnesses. A 1990 study of mortality in New York City's Harlem found that black men in that community were less likely to reach the age of 65 than were men in Bangladesh'' (*27*).

Being poor in a prosperous society is associated with frustration, boredom, and despair — crippling states of mind that undermine stable relationships and family life, and lead some to seek escape in drugs. In the industrialized world, injecting drug use is a dominant factor in the picture of AIDS. But a closer look shows that the risk is not confined to injecting behaviour; drugs play a wider and more complex role. For example, ''crack'' cocaine (a smokable form of cocaine) is strongly associated with the spread of HIV in some communities, as demonstrated by a 1989 study in the South Bronx area of New York City, where investigators found that nearly one in three crack users, who were heterosexual and did not inject drugs, were HIV-positive (*24*).

Alcohol, too, plays a powerful and prob-

Poverty as a bar to care

In Addis Ababa's Armed Forces Hospital, a young man with HIV-related tuberculosis is dying a slow, agonizing death. The only drug available for his condition in the hospital dispensary has elicited an allergic reaction causing him to shed most of his skin, and his body now weeps like a giant wound. His breathing is fast and shallow, his eyes are closed, and the nurses have no pain-killer on hand to ease his suffering.

In many hospitals in developing countries, kindness and compassion from the staff are all that is on offer to people with AIDS, for drugs of any kind are in short supply or simply unavailable. But even this level of care is beyond the reach of a large proportion of sick people. Most hospitals in the developing world are in towns and cities, while rural areas are served by clinics with even less satisfactory supplies and services. Thus people with AIDS — as with any other disease — often go without the simple medicines that could ease their pain or bring down a fever, let alone the more powerful drugs needed to cure an opportunistic infection or prolong life.

The problem is not confined to developing countries. A 1990 report from the US National Commission on AIDS revealed that 29% of people with AIDS in the USA have no health care insurance whatsoever, meaning they must pay for their own treatment, try to get care in a government hospital, or, all too often, go without.

"Once I went to a hospital in New York City. They asked me if I had Medicaid [government health insurance]. When they found out I didn't have Medicaid they didn't want to help me," said Ralph Hernandez. "The nurse said: 'Oh, your sores don't look that bad, I've seen worse.' My legs hurt so bad I couldn't walk without the crutches I had stolen. They didn't even clean my sores, they just gave me antibiotics and put me out on the street to clean them myself. Now, how am I going to keep my sores clean when I'm living in the subway ditch? You know how they are going to stay? Dirty" (3).

Health coverage in other industrialized countries is fortunately much more complete, but the poor everywhere are less well served than others in the population. Poor mothers, for example, often do not go to the doctor or into hospital when they need to, simply because they cannot afford to pay anyone to look after their children. In general, people living in poverty tend to be less aware of when to seek care, and less sure of how to work the system — especially if they are ill-educated or immigrants with little grasp of the host country's language.

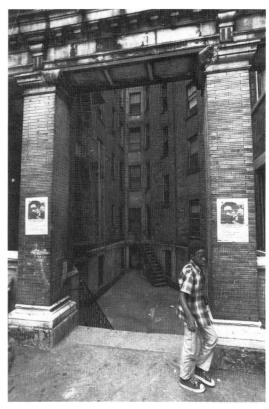

The lives of many African-Americans are marked by poverty and discrimination, which are risk factors for AIDS. They suffer from disproportionate levels of HIV infection.

ably underestimated role in the spread of AIDS. Like other drugs, it dispels inhibitions and impairs judgement, which can result in unintended forms of sexual behaviour. In addition, sex is frequently negotiated — for fun or for money — in the same places as alcohol, whether it be a party, night-club or bar.

Many of the daily problems experienced by poor people are compounded by low self-esteem and fatalism bred of powerlessness. These attitudes, too, have implications for AIDS prevention, because people who feel they have no future — youngsters who have seen nothing but broken homes, joblessness and want, or people confronted daily with hunger and disease — tend to wonder why they should take precautions against, or even care about, a distant threat like AIDS.

Child prostitution: a universal tragedy

Despite laws in most countries explicitly banning the prostitution of minors, countless children — some not yet teenagers — are reportedly working in brothels or on the streets.

Child prostitution appears to have been given a boost by clients' fears of AIDS. Pimps and middle-men play on men's fears by stressing the ''innocence'' and virginal qualities of young prostitutes, which suggest they are more likely to be infection-free. But for the children themselves the dangers are great. The immature genital tract of young girls is thought to be extra susceptible to HIV infection, especially when ruptured by forced sex. And anal sex, to which young boys particularly will be subjected, is a high-risk practice because of the tearing of the tissues.

It is impossible to know exactly how many youngsters are caught up in this illegal and secretive trade. But recent studies by the United Nations Educational, Scientific and Cultural Organization (UNESCO) on countries in Africa, Asia and Latin America revealed that child prostitution is extremely common. And in Europe and North America, too, under-age prostitutes are estimated to number in the hundreds of thousands (*28*).

The trade in children is international. Thus, youngsters from Bangladesh and India reportedly end up in brothels in the eastern Mediterranean; Burmese and Chinese youngsters in brothels in Thailand; and young Thais and Filipinas in the brothels of Europe.

Many are sold by their parents to middle-men who pretend to be recruiting workers for restaurants, carpet factories, or domestic service — occupations which would be damaging enough to the mental and physical health of the very young. But frequently it is the parents themselves who offer their children to customers for sex. At a 1993 conference organized by UNESCO on ''the sex trade and human rights'', Dr Duong Quynh Hoa, director of a paediatric hospital in Viet Nam's Ho Chi Minh City, reported seeing many sexually abused children brought for treatment by their fathers. She described one 12-year-old ''as bleeding from her wounds and as torn as if she had given birth. [Her father] told me: 'We've earned $300, so it's enough. She can stop'.''

One parent, challenged by the doctor about the dangers he was exposing his daughter to, replied simply that she had not yet entered puberty, and so could not get pregnant. ''And anyway,'' he told the doctor, ''once she has a packet of money, she'll be sure to find a husband willing to overlook her past'' (*29*).

CHAPTER 15

Women, sex and AIDS

"To enable women to protect themselves there are three issues at stake: improving the social and economic status of women; providing a method over which they have sufficient control; or getting more men to adopt safer sex. This is not an academic exercise in setting priorities, but a question of life and death for many women." — *Dr Eka Esu Williams, Nigeria (30)*

The recreation hall is packed as the City Healthworkers' Acting Troupe presents a drama about AIDS to a thousand migrant workers who have come from all over southern Africa to dig gold in the Transvaal. On stage the man strikes his wife for daring to suggest that he wear a condom during sex. Suddenly — and to the consternation of the cast, who expected the opposite reaction — the audience erupts in cheers and waving fists.

The scene illustrates one of the most intractable barriers to the control of AIDS: the subordination and powerlessness of women. For many women, the simple message of most education campaigns to "love carefully, stick to one faithful partner or use a condom" means little. A host of cultural, legal, and economic factors limit the control they have over their lives, their sexual relationships, and their ability to protect themselves from infection.

In some parts of the world, it is unacceptable for "good" women to take the initiative in sexual relationships — so unacceptable that many dare not bring up the subject of safe sex even with their regular, committed partners. To do so is to risk being rejected, beaten up, or even thrown out by men on whom, in many cases, they are completely dependent for economic survival and social status.

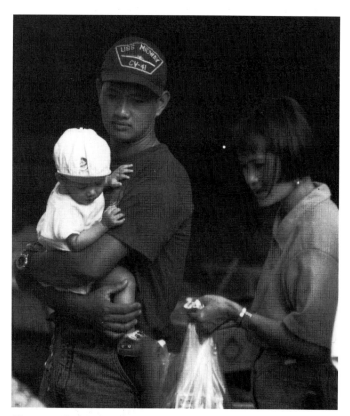

Men as well as women are trapped by the social and cultural conventions that require women to be subservient. They both need to be freed from the constraints of their social conditioning and helped towards a fairer — and less dangerous — relationship with one another.

Monogamy for whom?

There are some cultures in which casual sex is tolerated for neither partner in a marriage, others in which it is tolerated for both. In most cultures, however, women are expected to remain faithful to their husbands, while it is acceptable, even traditional, for men to have more than one sex partner, even though this often contradicts the prevailing moral code. The wives are supposed to tolerate their husbands' infidelity, but since AIDS entered the picture, the price of this tolerance has been raised inestimably.

In country after country, women report feelings of helplessness over their partners' extramarital behaviour, and their own vulnerability to AIDS. In Uganda, a researcher found that nearly one-third of the women she interviewed believed themselves to be at risk of HIV infection because they could neither control the extramarital affairs of their partners nor bring up the subject of condoms (*18*). In Belize, two-thirds of the women interviewed felt the same way. And in Jamaica, a woman told researchers: "The chances are that as a woman you are

> *All the gender issues we had never tackled came up at once"*, says Theresa Kaijage, a founding member of the Tanzanian AIDS service organization called WAMATA. *"Initially we ignored them or thought they were irrelevant. We thought it was Eurocentric to tackle them in Africa, because we thought our African culture was different and dealt with things in a different way. All the agendas that we had ignored — legal, educational and health problems, inequitable gender relations — suddenly we are dealing with these multiple issues, which people have not learned to analyse in a way that promotes equal sharing of both resources and power at all levels. In order to deal with AIDS, we have had to confront these"* (*32*).

going to get AIDS because your man has had sex with someone with HIV and brings it home to you. How can you protect yourself? By insisting that the man uses a condom? He has the power. He says he's not doing it. So what next? For far too many of us it boils down to either no sex and therefore no support system for yourself and your children, or the risk of contracting AIDS" (*31*).

A woman may know her partner is sleeping with other women, but she is likely to be drawn into an elaborate charade to protect his reputation and self-esteem at the expense of her safety. The situation is tellingly described by Refiloe Serote of Alexandra AIDS Action in South Africa, but it could just as well describe many other cultures. "For example, a situation like this develops: if your man comes home at 3 a.m. smelling of a perfume you don't recognize, that's the time he's going to ask for sex because he's trying to clear his conscience by making you think he hasn't already had it. But if he goes out drinking with the boys, he comes home and goes straight to sleep peacefully. You have to go along with whatever he asks, even if you're smelling this strange perfume, because you can't say 'no'."

The risk to monogamous women is due not only to their partners' relations with other women. Some men who do not consider themselves homosexual or even bisexual — and who

may even be married and have children — have sex with other men as well as with women.

In some cases this homosexual activity is situational, i.e., it occurs in situations such as confinement in prisons, on military bases, and in migrant labour camps, where men are segregated from women for long periods of time. In other cases, men who consider themselves heterosexual have occasional sexual contact with other men. And in some countries, men who would prefer to be exclusively homosexual, but who are afraid to do so openly, succumb to the social pressure to marry and have children, but have relationships with men at the same time, sometimes secretly.

In countries where injecting drug use occurs, women may be at risk from their partners' needle-sharing with other drug users rather than their sexual behaviour. Numerous studies have found that such men are often unwilling to use condoms with their female sex partners, many of whom do not inject drugs.

Feelings of powerlessness and inhibitions about broaching the subject of risk or negotiating condom use are universal. "[Even] the life-threatening nature of AIDS may not be sufficient to overcome them, but may simply increase the anxiety levels of women," commented a psychologist.

It is worth noting, however, that in every country, there are some women in relationships in which sex is engaged in with care and concern for both partners. In a community where 30% of women feel they have no control, a large proportion of women presumably

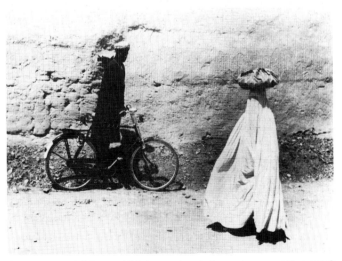

In some parts of the world, it is a major challenge to ensure that AIDS information reaches all women.

feel they *do* have some control. The challenge is to find out what makes the difference, and to use the insights to help those who are the most powerless.

To have a child or not

The issue of safe sex can present women with another painful dilemma. In many parts of the world fertility is a paramount value, and a woman's only path to social status and self-fulfilment is through childbearing. But in the AIDS era, and particularly in communities with high levels of HIV infection, women find themselves caught between the conflicting need to protect themselves against infection and the desire — indeed, the social imperative — to have children. In essence this means they are faced with a lonely and agonizing choice between physical survival and social acceptance.

Women get the blame

Paradoxically, since time immemorial women have been blamed for the spread of sexually transmitted diseases. Among certain peoples in Thailand and Uganda, STDs are known as "women's diseases" (*18*). And in Swahili, the lingua franca of much of east Africa, the word for STD means, literally, "disease of woman". By a cruel and irrational irony, single and educated Ugandan women — whose independence is seen by some men as a threat to the status quo — are being blamed for AIDS. "The tendency ... to scapegoat women who stand outside the structure of female subordination is an important issue in Ugandan society," write sociologists Tony Barnett and Piers Blaikie (*25*).

Essays on HIV/AIDS written by Ugandan schoolchildren show how deep the prejudice goes. In their writings, 40 youngsters expressed the opinion that women were mainly responsible for spreading HIV, while only three named men. These views were held by girls as well as boys, highlighting the tendency of the "victims" of prejudice to accept its assumptions as natural (*25*).

In particular, female prostitutes have, almost universally, been characterized as "vec-

WHO estimates that over 13 million women will have become infected with HIV by the year 2000.

tors of disease" — a description that completely ignores the role played by the customer, and that is strikingly never applied to men, no matter how high their levels of infection.

Even people infected by other routes blame prostitutes. In the USA, many men diagnosed with AIDS first blamed their infection on a female prostitute. Only when interviewed at length did they admit to injecting drugs or having sex with men.

The harsh judgement extends even to women who are sick. "[If you have AIDS] society rejects you. When you die you will not even be missed because you have died of a shameful disease," a married woman in Zaire told researchers. "They will say that this woman has strayed. They will not see that maybe she has remained faithful while her husband has strayed. Given the status of women in most... societies AIDS is doubly stigmatizing for women" (*33*).

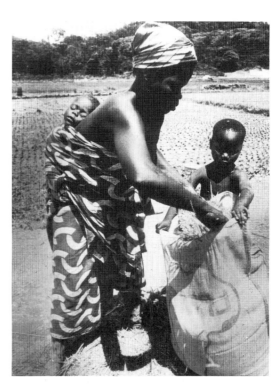

In many countries, a woman's only path to social status and self-fulfilment is through childbearing. Where levels of HIV infection are high, women may find themselves caught between the conflicting needs to avoid exposure to the virus and to become pregnant.

This stigma encourages women who know or suspect they might be infected to avoid finding out, hide their status if they do get tested, and delay seeking the professional help and treatment they so badly need. It also makes it doubly difficult for them to bring up the subject of safe sex and condoms with their partners, even to protect the partner from infection.

Sex and survival

It is not coincidental that the countries in which the virus is now spreading fastest heterosexually are generally those in which women's status is low.

Wherever sex discrimination leaves women undereducated, unskilled, unable to gain title to land or other vital resources in their own names, and low in self-esteem, it also leaves them especially vulnerable to HIV infection. Their access to vital information about the virus is limited, as is their choice of livelihood, and in hard times many find it necessary to trade sex for money, food or shelter.

> " For women, the reform of laws governing socio-economic status which can empower them to influence their husband's behaviour and also to mean 'no' to unwanted and unprotected sex when they say so is very urgent. What are we doing about our laws relative to rape, legal status of women, inheritance, etc?" — *Lesotho AIDS bulletin (34)*

Researchers from the University of Addis Ababa investigating the social background to prostitution in Ethiopia found that the great majority of women they questioned had little or no education. Many had married and struggled to cope with the adult responsibilities of motherhood and home-making before reaching their teens. The women came predominantly from the rural north where poverty, drought, famine and civil war have crushed communities and scattered families. Arriving without skills in the towns and cities, they had gone into prostitution as the only real alternative to destitution.

In Pattaya, a small, bustling resort on the Gulf of Thailand, the sex industry is clearly visible. At night there are few people on the beach, for what attracts most to Pattaya is in the bars and massage parlours. Here, under flashing ultraviolet lights, women dance to loud music, near-naked on raised stages, as customers sit round on bar stools drinking beer and searching out likely sex partners.

Behind the scenes all hint of glamour quickly evaporates, for here, in tiny locker-rooms, the young women are packed together in sweltering tropical heat, waiting their turn on stage. Most are from poor rural areas and have little education and few marketable skills. They are people like "Noi", a young woman with bright intelligent eyes and hair curling around an oval face. Left by her husband when their child was still a baby, she was unable to earn enough money with her own small business of making and selling sweets to support herself and her son, or to discharge the cultural obligation she has, as a daughter, to provide for her parents. "It was my own choice to become a prostitute — no one forced me," she said. "But the alternative was poverty. I make first-class sweets, but I have no other training. My desire now is to build my parents a good house and then to get out of this business for good," and she spreads her hands in a gesture of finality.

On the other side of the world, in Zimbabwe, six women tell of the pressures that led them to prostitution, including drought and other natural disasters, the inheritance system in their countries which deprives women of land and resources when their husbands die, and general poverty. "When poor women must choose between immediate economic crisis in their households versus the possibility of a dimly understood disease, the choice is easy," commented one observer (33).

Women who go into sex work are often extremely vulnerable to HIV infection. They may know nothing about the virus or how to protect themselves, and the laws and stigmas associated with prostitution may make it difficult for them to acknowledge what they are doing or to seek out more experienced prostitutes to teach them how to work safely. But even if they are well informed, they are apt to find it hard to insist on safe sexual practices because of fears that a client unwilling to use a condom will go elsewhere. Furthermore, in many coun-

■ A woman in Manila, Philippines, put in a nutshell the dilemma faced by so many women like herself across the world: "AIDS might make me sick one day," she said. "But if I don't work my family would not eat and we would all be sick anyway" (*24*).

tries, simply carrying condoms can be taken by police as evidence that a woman is a prostitute.

Besides economic desperation, there are other forces at work in the relationship between prostitution and the subordination of women. In many societies low status means that women are not free to choose their own lifestyles; standards of sexual behaviour imposed on them by society are much stricter than those on men, and women who deviate from those standards are heavily stigmatized. Under these circumstances, any woman who has sex outside marriage — for whatever reason — does so at the expense of her reputation and social standing. She joins, almost automatically, an "underclass" of women who are looked down upon by other women as well as by men, who nevertheless rely on them for the satisfaction of their sexual needs.

In Ethiopia, for example, virginity in an unmarried woman is so highly valued, says Professor Mekonnen Bishaw, that young girls in traditional communities never mix socially with boys, and dating and dances are unheard of. However, such chastity is not expected of young men, and many have their first sexual experience with a prostitute — a practice which is not openly condoned, but understood, accepted, and very common.

To a certain extent these double standards for sexuality exist in all societies. But where the distinction between "good women who won't" and "bad women who will" is most marked, the "bad women" are among the most vulnerable to HIV infection in the world. And the lower their status, the higher their vulnerability, as many surveys of HIV infection rates show.

For example, a study of female prostitutes in the USA found the highest infection rates among street prostitutes, who, for the most part, came from poor black or Hispanic communities. The lowest infection rates were among escort service and brothel workers, most of whom were middle class and white.

Similarly, researchers in Kenya found that prostitutes from the lower socioeconomic classes, who were paid an average of 50 US cents per transaction, were twice as likely to be infected as women from the upper end of the market, who earned up to 30 times as much per transaction and had many fewer customers per year (*35*). And surveys in Thailand in 1992 found HIV prevalence rates of 35% among women working in low-charge brothels serving local clients, compared with rates of up to 17% among women employed in bars and other places of entertainment. The woman's risk grows with the likelihood that her clients and other sex partners are infected, and that she herself will be too poor, too rushed, or too desperate to insist on safe sex.

Among the most vulnerable sex workers are women who travel across state and national boundaries to find work. In a strange community, often confronted with a strange language, they have more difficulty negotiating with clients and with the managers of the places where they work. And if they are in the country illegally, facing the risk of prison sentences and deportation, they are even more powerless.

Travel is, in fact, a central feature of prostitution. Young women from Myanmar cross the border into Thailand on one-day passes looking for work, sometimes under the auspices of brokers who recruit women to work in the brothels along the border and may force them to stay against their will. Estonian women fly to Helsinki or Stockholm for the weekend, contact clients in major tourist hotels, and return home with hard currency. Czech and Hungarian women take the bus to Vienna on Friday, work that night, shop on Saturday with the hard currency they earn, and return home on Saturday night. And women from the Philippines arrange passages to Hamburg with corrupt travel agencies that specialize in international work migration, only to find themselves caught, without proper documentation, in a trap of debts which they can hope to pay off only through work in brothels.

Sex tourism is another aspect of the exploitation of impoverished women, though the promoters of this hugely lucrative industry do their best to cover the reality of the prostitutes' lives behind a façade of exoticism and social sanction. It is also a further demonstration of double standards, as men from the rich world, or from countries where extramarital sex brings harsh penalties, travel great distances to find sex partners. Though some will be lonely and socially inadequate men looking for an intimacy that they have failed to find at home, many are intent upon finding partners who will make none of the emotional demands of wives or girlfriends in their own countries.

Besides overt prostitution, sex is used as a bargaining chip in a number of other survival strategies. In countries where men are expected to provide for all of their children, a woman without employment options may have children with several different men who are then duty-bound, by culture or law, to support her and her family. In this situation, of course, her need to bear children for economic survival conflicts with the need to protect herself from HIV infection.

Sometimes adolescent girls look for older — and often married — men of means, "sugar daddies", who can provide them with school fees or other necessities, and perhaps the odd luxury they could never afford. This may be the only way a girl from a poor family can hope to pay her way through school in countries where secondary schooling is not free. If the girl gets pregnant, however, she is likely to leave school, and if rejected by her family, may turn to prostitution to survive.

For many girls and women round the world, in fact, sex is the currency in which they are expected to pay for every opportunity in life, from gaining admission to overcrowded classes

> In Africa, boys who need to find their own school fees are more likely to engage in petty trade, buying things cheaply and selling them at inflated prices," says Dr Samuel Kalibala, GPA's counselling specialist. "The boys are regarded as clever and street-wise, but this wouldn't be acceptable for girls, who are brought up to see their attractiveness to men as their main asset."

in school, to passing exams, securing employment, being granted a trading licence in the local marketplace, keeping a job as a domestic servant, or even crossing a border. But AIDS has transformed what appeared to be strategies of survival into strategies of death, for women in such situations can do little to protect themselves from infection.

The AIDS epidemic demonstrates as clearly as any other modern issue that the subordination of women is more than a question of fundamental injustice to one half of society. It stifles discussion between sex partners without which safe sex is unlikely to happen. By creating conditions in which women find it hard to avoid the risk of infection, sex discrimination raises the general level of HIV infection within the community and increases the AIDS threat for *everyone*.

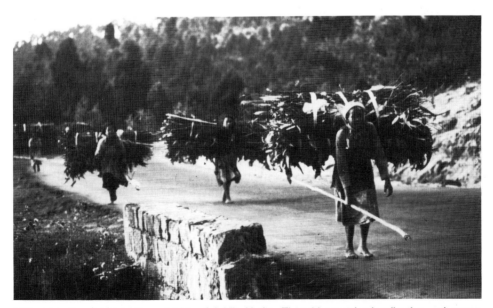

Women gather wood on the outskirts of Addis Ababa. The widespread subordination and powerlessness of women is one of the driving forces behind the spread of HIV, while the need to care for family members with AIDS has added a new burden to their already heavy workload.

PART IV

What can be done about AIDS?

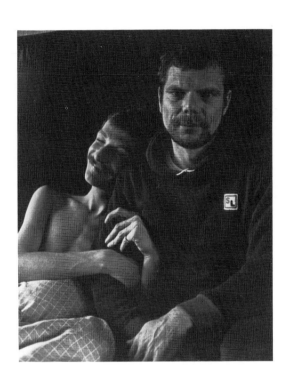

CHAPTER 16

Fighting back

"To care is a duty; to prevent is a responsibility. Prevention and care are the twin engines that should drive our effort for the containment of AIDS." — *Professor V. Ramalingaswami, India (36)*

Unlike other epidemic diseases such as cholera or measles, HIV infection does not cause sudden, widespread death, but remains hidden for years after it begins to spread. This characteristic, coupled with the fact that AIDS involves behaviour that many societies condemn, has been a great obstacle to setting up programmes to fight the epidemic. In the early days, too, the general debate about AIDS was mired in confusion, blame, prejudice and fear that tended to paralyse governments.

However, with strong advocacy from individuals and groups around the world — and assistance from WHO and other international agencies — virtually every country now has a functioning AIDS programme. (See tables in Annex for information on and from national programmes.) Most are guided by the objectives and principles of the global AIDS strategy (23).

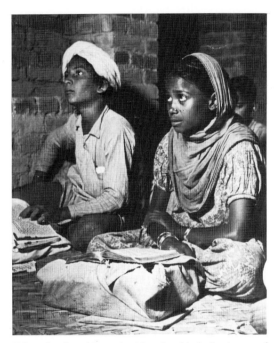

Education for girls, as in this school in India, is one of the main strategies for improving women's status and making them less vulnerable to HIV infection.

The umbrella: national AIDS programmes

The task of a national AIDS programme is threefold:

— to provide the policies, information campaigns, and health and social services that people need in order to protect themselves from HIV infection (see panel, next page);

— to meet the gradually expanding need for care as those who are infected with HIV go on to develop AIDS;

— to plan for and cope with the ripple effects of AIDS.

Above all, the national programme provides coordination and a technical support structure for all those who are working in the field. These include government officials from the health and other sectors (see Annex, Table 4), blood bank staff, nurses in primary health care clinics, members of the media and business communities, private individuals, and a wealth of nongovernmental organizations — some of them international, most at the grass roots of their own countries.

National programmes today are working on a wide range of activities, often in the face of constraints such as poverty, political instability and war. A good example of what is happening in many developing countries is provided by Malawi. One of the world's poorest nations, Malawi is host to hundreds of thousands of refugees from war-ravaged Mozambique, and is in the grip of one of the worst AIDS epidemics in Africa.

Here, the AIDS programme works through and with many different social and community organizations to deliver information, care and support to people at the grass roots. Women's groups and young people belonging to the Malawi Young Pioneers have received AIDS information and training in peer education. Muslim leaders have been trained in workshops on AIDS prevention and on the counselling of people with HIV infection or AIDS, and today the subject is discussed at Friday mosque meetings. Paramedics have been taught about AIDS prevention and enlisted to

Comprehensive prevention: what is it?

In the early days of the epidemic, national AIDS programmes and community groups seeking to stem the tide of HIV spread had no choice but to experiment. There was no way to know with certainty what prevention approaches would work best, especially for convincing people to change their sexual or drug-taking behaviour. And there was no guarantee that promoting condoms, say, or giving drug users clean injection equipment, would not somehow rebound and result in *more* rather than *less* unsafe behaviour.

Today, based on a decade of experience, we know that some prevention approaches work and others do not. What does *not* work is making people unduly fearful, or harassing them, or alienating them with threats of compulsory testing. What *does* work is to create a supportive social environment in which people can be informed about the whole range of options for safer behaviour, encouraged to assume responsibility for their own behaviour, and given the necessary social and health services support.

The current consensus is that a basic HIV prevention package includes at least the following:

• condom social marketing, that is, the promotion and distribution of condoms in the general population

• treatment of the conventional STDs, because of their role in facilitating HIV transmission

• AIDS education in schools to slow transmission to young people, who now account for about half of all HIV infections

• AIDS information through the mass media, aimed at the general population

• promotion of condom use by prostitutes and their clients

• maintenance of a safe blood supply

• needle-exchange programmes for injecting drug users.

There is now solid evidence that these prevention approaches reduce HIV transmission *without encouraging risk behaviour.* What is more, they can work in a matter of months, not the years or even decades once believed necessary for changing human behaviour.

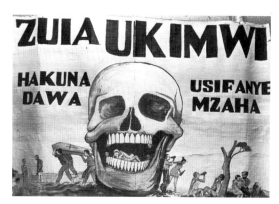

Many early AIDS information campaigns used fear to try to get people to change their sexual behaviour. But fear tactics proved counterproductive, encouraging prejudice and discrimination against people with AIDS instead of helpful behaviour change.

distribute condoms. And the business community has been drawn into the network with training courses in AIDS prevention and condom promotion.

The popular media also play an important role. Newspapers and radio programmes cover AIDS issues, making particular efforts to address fears and correct misconceptions; local choirs take part in AIDS song contests; popular musicians write and record music with AIDS themes; drama groups perform AIDS plays; and AIDS comics are produced for kids.

Besides showing ingenuity in spreading the word about AIDS, many countries have also demonstrated pragmatism in overcoming social conventions and mind-sets that are obstacles to the control of the epidemic. In Swaziland, for example, an organization called "Mantalk" attempts to open the dialogue between men and women on sexual matters. In Ethiopia, where a short while ago unmarried women were denied access to contraception, condoms are now available in a wide variety of outlets from bars and street kiosks to petrol stations. And in parts of Thailand, agreements worked out in discussions between the AIDS programme and police mean that drug users can attend treatment clinics without fear of arrest so long as they are not in possession of drugs: thus users are not forced underground where they are cut off from information and other HIV prevention services.

AIDS prevention is still very much a journey through uncharted territory, and programmes are changing and adapting in the light of experience all the time. For example, a number of countries — including Australia, Brazil and the United Kingdom — tried originally to instil fear as a way of encouraging people to change their behaviour. Posters and newspaper advertisements showed coffins being lowered into the ground, for example, or depicted death in the shape of the "Grim Reaper". But this quickly proved counterproductive, tending to increase stigma and kindle prejudice against infected people, rather than encouraging the as-yet-uninfected to take stock of their own behaviour. Besides, it had the effect of increasing anxiety in people who had little power to protect themselves.

Thailand, too, used fear in early campaigns to try to change behaviour. Posters showed close-up shots of some of the more visible and distressing opportunistic infections. But the focus changed in the light of experience. "Thailand's AIDS programme is very active, very alive, and very quick to learn and adapt as necessary," says Steve Kraus, GPA technical officer stationed in Bangkok. "It has become something of a university for the study of AIDS prevention in the region — practically every country has sent representatives here to observe how the Thai programme operates. The reason everyone knows about AIDS in Thailand is not that its epidemic or the behaviour behind it is unique, but that the country is much more open about it than some others in the region."

Moroccan Association Against AIDS *(Association marocaine de Lutte contre le SIDA,* ALCS) when she became aware of the cultural and religious constraints on the government programme. "There were certain aspects of AIDS prevention that could on no account be done by the Ministry of Health — in particular the work among female sex workers or among homosexuals. None of the groups with risk behaviour could be touched by a Ministry," she said. "For example, it is not yet admitted in Morocco that prostitution exists. People *know* it takes place, but its existence is not admitted officially."

She recognized, too, that stigmatized people are suspicious of government authorities and tend to reject any programme with an official stamp. She started ALCS in 1988 to disseminate information, encourage behaviour change, and offer care and support to people with HIV/AIDS. The organization is particularly committed to the protection of human rights and dignity and to fighting discrimination.

Among its many activities, ALCS produces leaflets, operates an AIDS helpline and runs free, anonymous testing centres. It also supports safer-sex programmes (including condom distribution) among female sex workers and gay and bisexual men. By showing respect for society's feelings and traditions, it has broken down some barriers to the preven-

"Grass-roots players"

As stated earlier, a vital — and, in some places, a dominant — role in national action against AIDS is played by nongovernmental organizations (NGOs). In many cases, they were first to respond to the distress of communities caught in the path of the epidemic, and often the only people prepared to speak up about AIDS.

"It is hard for a Ministry or for civil servants to work with populations which do not officially exist," says Dr Hakima Himmich, professor of medicine at the University of Casablanca, Morocco, who founded the first nongovernmental AIDS organization in the Maghreb.

Professor Himmich, who was a member of the national AIDS programme, started the

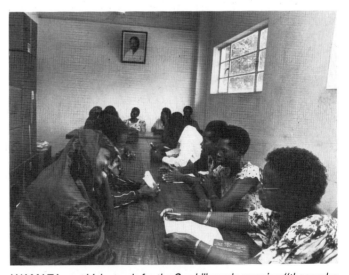

WAMATA — which stands for the Swahili words meaning "those who are in the front line" — was the first Tanzanian self-help organization for people with AIDS and their carers. Sharing experiences helps alleviate the isolation and stress that often threaten to overwhelm AIDS-affected families.

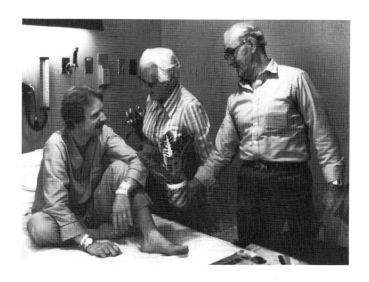

tion of AIDS in Morocco. Today, the Minister of Health is Honorary President of the association.

While this community initiative has been welcomed by the Moroccan Ministry of Health, some nongovernmental organizations operate in an atmosphere of official suspicion or indifference. But GPA's Deputy Director, Dr Dorothy Blake, stresses that close collaboration between national programmes and NGOs is essential to a strong campaign. ''The two have

AIDS patients are no different from people with other diseases. They need comfort and cheer.

NGOs take the lead

Nongovernmental organizations play an important role everywhere, but they are especially important in countries where government action is constrained by strong cultural or religious traditions. Among the many examples:

• *The Syrian Women's Union* plays an active part in raising awareness about HIV/AIDS, conducting seminars for health personnel, running workshops on education and counselling, and helping design information materials. Members of the Medical Services Office of the Union, in collaboration with the Ministry of Health, have also visited prisons and social work schools to give out information on AIDS and how to prevent it.

• *The Egyptian AIDS Society,* established in Alexandria in mid-1992 and funded largely by local businessmen, has talked about AIDS on television and held information days in universities, secondary schools and family planning centres. It has also organized information workshops for medical professionals, social workers and police officers. The society aims to give social and financial support to people with HIV infection and AIDS and their families, and to provide counselling to those who need it.

• *The Pakistan AIDS Prevention Society* was formed in 1990 by a group of people, including teachers and trade-unionists, who saw the need for broad-based community action. Its work is public information and education. Major objectives are to dispel prejudice, stigma and discrimination in a country where ignorance and denial of AIDS are still widespread.

• In 1992, the *Arab Scouts Movement,* a pan-Arab organization, brought together members from all national scout organizations for a meeting that focused, among other things, on AIDS. The meeting agreed that all national societies should provide their members with information on AIDS and how to protect oneself from the virus, so that they could spread the word among their families, friends and communities.

• In 1989 in Ljubljana, Slovenia, a group of drug users attending a psychotherapy programme threatened with closure, started *Stigma,* a self-help organization to look after the interests of drug users and give them information about AIDS. Despite public resistance and an uncertain relationship with the authorities — including the health services and

police — *Stigma* has established drop-in information centres for drug users in three towns. Volunteer staff offer advice and counselling, and the Ljubljana branch runs a needle-exchange programme. *Stigma* also operates telephone hotlines; publishes information materials and a newsletter; and takes advantage of any opportunity to campaign for the rights of drug users, and to promote safer drug injecting and sexual behaviour.

• *GAPA/RS* is an AIDS prevention programme for prisoners in the state of Rio Grande do Sul, Brazil. Its central activity has been the production of an educational comic book that incorporates AIDS information in the story of a man in prison. Six prisoners in Porto Alegre were involved in creating the story line and characters, so the comic has an authentic and credible voice, and conveys a positive image of prisoners. The comic raises issues of injecting drug use and unsafe sexual behaviour, and messages are reinforced by the inclusion of puzzles and quizzes for the reader. A condom is given away with each comic. The programme, which is to be adopted in other states, includes a video version of the story for showing in prisons.

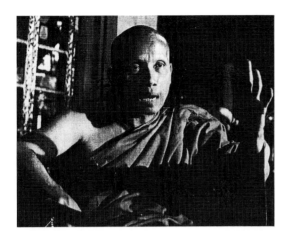

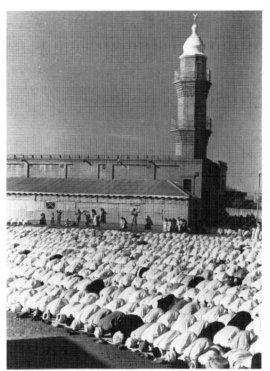

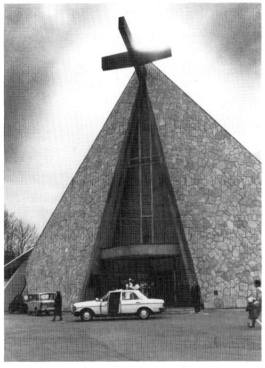

Because of their wide following and position of leadership in the community, religious leaders and congregations have a vital role to play in educating the public about AIDS and encouraging compassion for those affected by the epidemic. Many churches, mosques and temples are already involved in caring for AIDS patients and AIDS survivors.

complementary strengths. While governments have overall authority and can provide leadership and sometimes funds, NGOs are more in touch with communities at grassroots level,'' she says.

"Besides, many NGOs work in remote areas, so they are ideally placed to point out gaps and shortcomings in the provision of services. It also makes good sense to pool rather than to duplicate resources and effort.'' GPA promotes what it considers an invaluable partnership by encouraging national AIDS programmes to commit at least 15% of their budget to NGO activities.

> " No one who travels, visits communities, and talks to the grassroots players can fail to be struck by the demonstrations of courage, compassion and imagination that counterbalance prejudice and other mean-spirited reactions.''

Better tools in store?

Encouragement of behaviour change, condom promotion, STD care: the technology for HIV prevention is limited. And the medicines available for people who are already infected are woefully inadequate, for AIDS is still an incurable, fatal disease. Can we look to science for better tools for prevention and care?

When the first case of AIDS was recognized in 1981 the medical world was mystified. Yet within four years scientists had established that they were dealing with an infectious disease; they had isolated the causal virus, developed tests capable of detecting infection, and established the main routes of transmission. Never before has so much been learned about a new disease in so short a span of time.

An unprecedented effort continues to be made by biomedical researchers to uncover more of HIV's secrets, and to find a preventive vaccine and a cure. Meanwhile, social scientists are working to improve methods for helping people to achieve and sustain behaviour change in the difficult areas of sex and drug use.

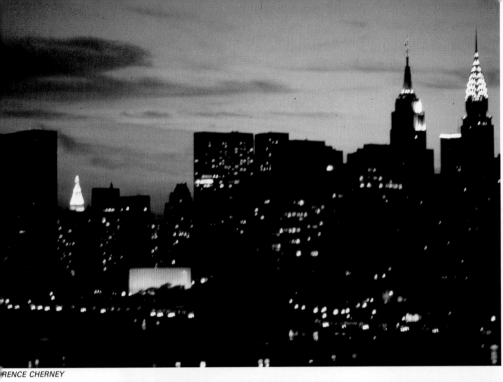

New York City, one of the epicentres of the AIDS epidemic in the USA.

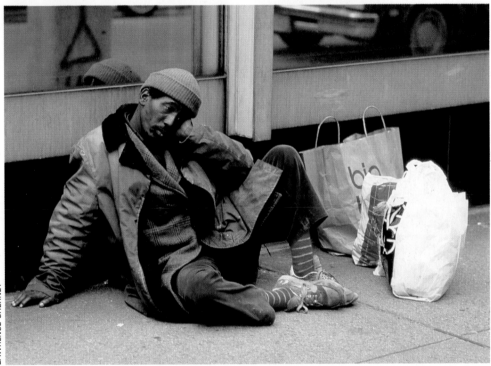

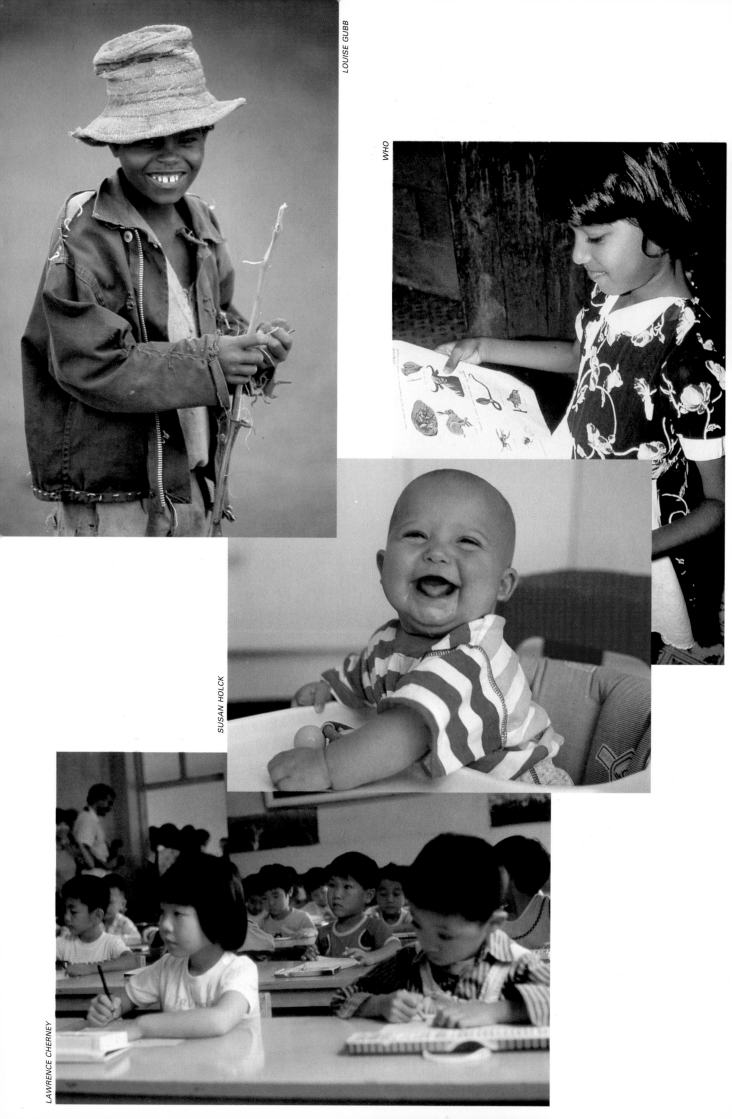

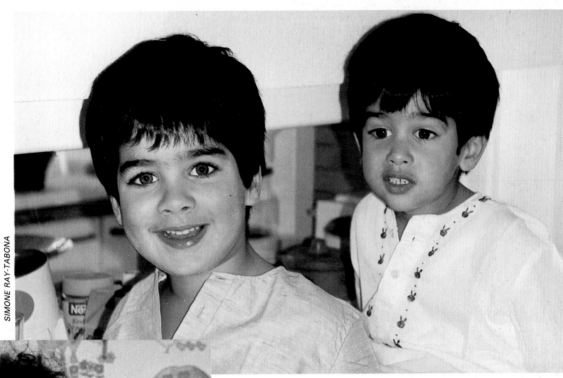

SIMONE RAY-TABONA

SUZANNE CHERNEY

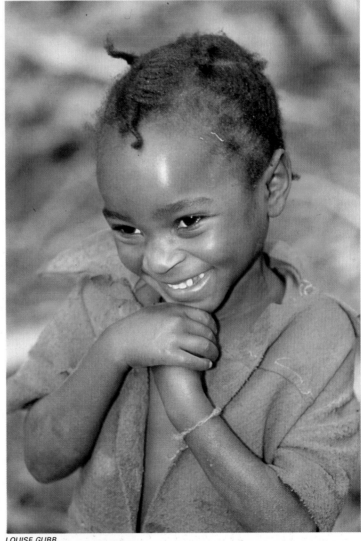

LOUISE GUBB

If children are to be protected from AIDS, it is essential that we start giving them the facts about the virus even before they become sexually active. They must not be allowed to die of ignorance.

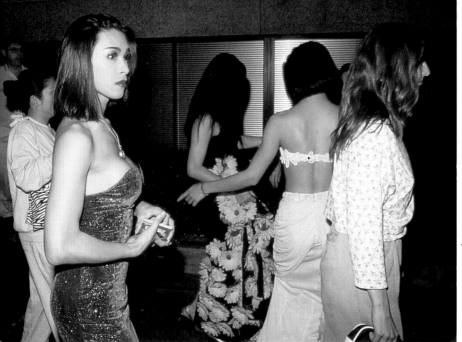

GÉRARD DIEZ

◄ This transvestite cabaret is a major tourist attraction, playing to full houses most nights.

In Ethiopia, sex workers at the lower end of the sex industry are among the most powerless and vulnerable to HIV. Working out of their own homes deprives them of the moral support they could get from colleagues and bar-owners in insisting on condom use by clients.
▼

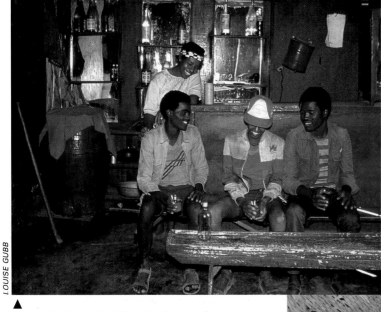

LOUISE GUBB

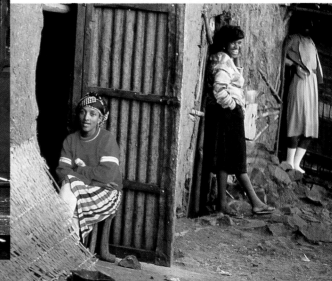

▲ A bar in Nazareth, Ethiopia. Among the country's 50 million people, the groups most heavily affected by AIDS are female prostitutes and their male clients.

LOUISE GUBB

GÉRARD DIEZ

Sex tourists with prostitutes. While most prostitution is a local phenomenon, involving local clients and sex workers, the movement of prostitutes and clients from country to country in search of partners is an international phenomenon. ►

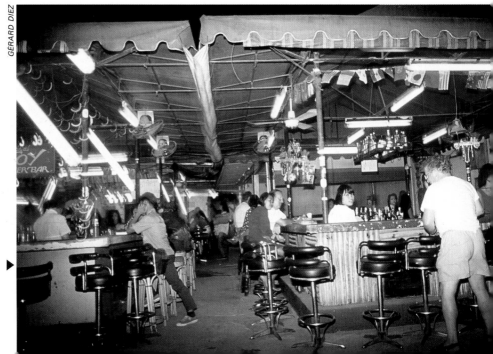

CHAPTER 17

The promise of science

"AIDS challenges our ethical and moral foundations as no disease has ever done. If we can build an ethic of caring into all our scientific thinking, our scientific work, our scientific enterprise, we will go that extra mile because we are one family." — *Dr Maxine Ankrah, USA/Ghana (37)*

Cure — and care

When scientists discovered in 1983 that the cause of AIDS was a virus, they realized that finding a cure would be extremely difficult. Bacterial infections are readily curable with antibiotics, fungus infections with antifungal drugs. But viruses multiply inside living cells, using the cell's own mechanism. An antiviral drug that interferes with the reproduction of the virus is likely to interfere with the normal cell's function as well, causing side-effects in the patient.

Working hard to overcome this obstacle, researchers have come up with several antiretroviral drugs (HIV is a member of the retrovirus family). While these do not destroy HIV, they slow down its reproduction and decrease the number of HIV-related symptoms and diseases, giving patients a better quality of life. However, the drugs may cause side-effects, and their therapeutic effects are temporary. Moreover, the antiretrovirals on the market today are extremely expensive, which limits their potential for use in developing countries.

Rather than cure, the best prospects in the short term are for improved care of people with HIV and AIDS. For while HIV infection itself is viral and hard to treat, many of the opportunistic infections to which seropositive people are prone are caused by bacteria, parasites and fungi, and can be treated or even prevented. For example, some drugs are effective against fungus infections of the mouth and throat, which if left untreated cause so much pain that patients are unable to eat and become malnourished. Other drugs can treat and prevent tuberculosis and pneumonia.

While these treatments can do much to alleviate the suffering caused by HIV-related illness, they — like drugs for many other ailments — are simply unaffordable in many parts of the developing world. For example, the drugs needed for a fungal infection of the mouth cost up to US$10 for initial treatment and $1 to $7 a

week thereafter for maintenance, while those needed for a fungal infection of the oesophagus cost around $30, and $2–7 a week for maintenance. A full course of therapy for tuberculosis ranges in cost from $40 to $75.

To the problem of lack of cash is added that of access: drugs often do not reach those in need of them. In some cases they are not on the "essential drugs list" — a basic list of medicines for which special pricing, funding and delivery arrangements exist for developing countries. Or the drugs may be in stock in hospitals or clinics that are simply out of reach for many rural people, or that are staffed by health workers lacking the necessary experience or skills to care for people with AIDS.

Clearly, the different obstacles involved need to be tackled one by one. On drug costs, WHO, the United Nations Development Programme (UNDP) and representatives of the pharmaceutical companies have begun discussions with a view to seeing how medicines for developing countries might be made appropriate and affordable. One topic under discussion is the possibility of developing pricing mechanisms that might bring more products within reach of developing countries. Another goal is to simplify licensing procedures so that drugs

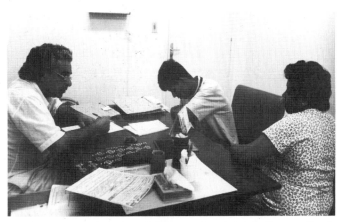

A person with HIV and his mother consult a doctor in Santos, Brazil. Though there is no cure for AIDS, there are drugs to treat opportunistic infections. Much can be done to relieve pain and suffering and prolong life.

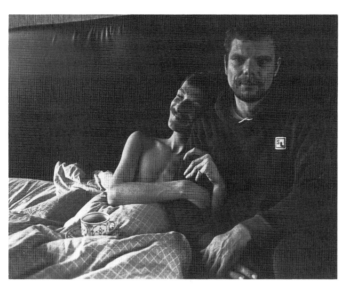

The idea of a "buddy" service is to pair each person with AIDS with a "buddy" — a volunteer who visits, hugs and helps out. Such services, pioneered in many countries by gay organizations, can bring enrichment to both people.

do not have to go through lengthy and expensive tests in one country after another.

Working with countries, WHO is trying to ensure that essential drugs lists are updated to meet the emerging needs of people with HIV infection and AIDS. In addition, guidelines have been developed for the clinical management of adults and children with HIV infection. The guidelines set out step-by-step plans for treatment and diagnosis according to the patient's signs and symptoms, and can be used by health workers at three different levels of health care facilities.

Preparing the ground for vaccine trials

While virus infections are difficult to cure, they have traditionally been good candidates for prevention through vaccines. Smallpox, eradicated thanks to a vaccine, was a virus infection, and so are measles and polio — fatal diseases against which most of the world's children are now immunized.

But early hopes of developing an HIV vaccine gave way to deepening doubt as scientists realized they were up against an extremely complicated virus, which changes constantly and varies strikingly from one part of the world to the next.

"Smallpox is very stable; there is only one type of the virus, so the vaccine developed against it was effective everywhere in the world," says Dr José Esparza, chief of vaccine development at GPA. "Influenza is less stable. The virus often changes every year, which means that a vaccine effective in one epidemic period is not necessarily effective in the next. But though influenza changes over time, it's basically the same virus all over the world. HIV is much more complicated because it varies both temporally and geographically. So we have many different virus strains — all of them evolving — in different parts of the world."

Development of an HIV vaccine has also been stymied by the unusual immune system reaction to infection with this virus (see panel, page 6) and the lack of a good animal model in which to test candidate vaccines. Chimpanzees — to date, the only animals of potential use in HIV vaccine development — are a rare and expensive species, and their use in scientific research is controversial.

Despite these obstacles, a number of candidate vaccines have passed the preclinical phase of trials, including studies of their safety in animals, and have entered small clinical trials in humans. Only large-scale efficacy trials, involving several hundreds or thousands of volunteers, will show if these vaccines really protect people against HIV infection.

Because of the great variability in HIV strains, vaccine trials will have to be conducted not only in industrialized countries but in the developing world. Steps are being taken in collaboration with WHO to ensure that at least four countries — Brazil, Rwanda, Thailand and Uganda — are ready to join the global vaccine development effort and begin large-scale trials just as soon as safe and appropriate candidate vaccines are available. These sites were selected by an international committee of experts who were seeking:

- study populations with a high incidence of HIV infection, who have the most to gain from successful vaccine development;
- relatively settled populations, because of the need for regular and long-term follow-up of trial participants;
- populations with relatively well-developed health and laboratory facilities;
- locations where there would be popular and political support for trials.

To ensure that the chosen locations will be able to cope with the vaccine trials, WHO has begun to strengthen their infrastructure, by upgrading health and research facilities and training local scientists as necessary. A worldwide network of laboratories has also been set up to isolate local HIV strains for use in vaccine and drug research. Trials conducted at these sites will have to conform to the highest ethical standards, respecting volunteers' individual rights and community traditions. Intensive health education, including the distribution of condoms, will continue throughout the trials — even though this may slow down research findings.

But it is unwise to expect a quick end to the HIV epidemic with a vaccine. Even if efficacy trials are launched by the mid-1990s, a vaccine cannot realistically be on the market before the year 2000. And at best a vaccine will only complement other prevention methods. For one thing, vaccine programmes take a long time to reach most or all of the target population. It took national immunization programmes close to two decades to achieve global coverage rates of 80% with BCG and vaccines against diphtheria, whooping cough, tetanus and measles — and, unlike an HIV vaccine, these did not have to be developed from scratch. Another issue is that no HIV vaccine is likely to be 100% effective. As AIDS is a fatal disease, vaccinated people will probably want and need to use other means of protection as well.

In other words, there is no getting round the fact that prevention efforts will have to continue to rely on safer sex (through behaviour change and the use of condoms and other barriers to HIV) and prompt, effective treatment for conventional STDs.

New focus on the conventional STDs

The now clear link between the rapid spread of HIV infection and the presence of other STDs (see Chapter 3) has focused attention on a badly neglected public health problem. Every year, at least 250 million infections other than HIV are transmitted through unprotected sexual intercourse, yet the control of STDs carries a low priority in most of the world. Treatment facilities are often inadequate and unwelcoming, and the stigma connected with STD makes many people reluctant to acknowledge symptoms and seek treatment. This is particularly true of women, even though their complications tend to be more severe than those in men — pelvic inflammatory disease, infertility, and ectopic pregnancy, which can be fatal.

Status of national STD programmes, 1992*

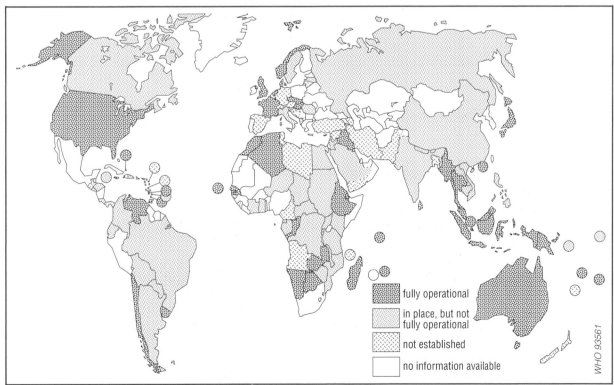

fully operational

in place, but not fully operational

not established

no information available

WHO 93561

* Based on answers by countries to a GPA questionnaire.

Besides, many STDs — again, especially in women — are relatively symptom-free in the early stages, so that people are unaware they are infected.

While the conventional STDs facilitate the transmission of HIV, HIV can make these STDs harder to treat because of immune suppression. So there is a new urgency to the task of controlling STDs. Fortunately, many measures aimed at prevention — education and information, promotion of condoms and other safer sex practices — are the same for both HIV and the conventional STDs. And the target audiences are identical. WHO is therefore encouraging STD programmes and AIDS prevention programmes to cooperate, or even merge in some cases.

There are still major hurdles, including making STD services more user-friendly, and motivating people to seek early treatment. But one problem may now be solved. "Up to now it was said that you needed laboratory tests to diagnose STDs in women. But there are countries where there is not a single laboratory which can do that," says Dr Peter Piot, GPA's Associate Director who is in charge of STDs. "So we have come up with a method for diagnosis based on just asking a few questions and doing some examination. For example, a recent change of sex partner raises an individual's risk of infection enormously. By eliciting information which gives you a risk profile, and by doing a simple examination, you can get a reasonably accurate diagnosis."

Protection methods women can control

Experience of the past five to ten years has confirmed that women are less able than men to protect themselves from the sexual transmission of HIV because condom use requires — at the very least — cooperation from men.

Proper STD care should go some way towards reducing women's vulnerability, but science holds out other hopes as well. Efforts are under way to develop "barrier methods" that can be used by women when they are unable to get their partner to use a condom, or when they otherwise wish to control the prevention process.

The "female condom" — essentially a pouch that women insert into the vagina before intercourse — is now on the market in a few developed countries. Initial studies suggest that it is acceptable in some settings to women at high risk of HIV infection, such as prostitutes. Though the female condom has been developed and recommended for contraception, studies will soon be conducted to determine its effectiveness in preventing STDs. Another issue is that the female condom is expensive and has been approved for single use only. Research is under way to find out if it continues to be effective if washed and reused.

A further drawback of the female condom is its visibility. There is an urgent need to find barrier methods that women can apply, if necessary, without their partner's knowledge.

Spermicides are one possibility. Intravaginal spermicides have been used as a female-controlled method of contraception for the past few decades. Because they also have antimicrobial properties, these products likewise decrease the risk of acquiring some STDs and they have been shown, at least in test-tubes, to inactivate HIV. The drawback is that spermicides, especially when used several times a day (as in sex work), have been found to cause vaginal irritation, and this might actually increase the risk of HIV transmission. A top research priority for WHO is determining the safety and protective efficacy of existing spermicides, and developing a non-irritating product that will protect against HIV infection and other STDs — perhaps even one without spermicidal activity, for women who wish to conceive a child.

Societies under the microscope

With prevention riding above all on behaviour change, social scientists are conducting research to find out the best ways of achieving this.

"In the early days of the epidemic, we were severely handicapped by a lack of basic information about patterns of sexual behaviour and patterns of injecting drug use, but much has been learned since then," says Dr Peter Aggleton, chief of social and behavioural studies for GPA. "In a way, AIDS made it legitimate to study sexuality and sexual behaviour. A great deal has been learned in only a few years. We now know that sexual behaviour is considerably more diverse than was imagined before. Homosexual as well as heterosexual behaviour, for example, is present in all societies and is part of the normal repertoire of human sexual expression. By accepting and using this diversity as our starting point, we can plan more effective interventions.''

Behavioural research has also examined the ways in which individuals understand themselves — as opposed to how society might define them. For example, in many parts of the world it is common to receive gifts and perhaps money in exchange for sex, yet only sometimes do the women and men concerned consider themselves prostitutes. More commonly, to receive such favours is simply a way of life. Prevention strategies that make erroneous assumptions about how people see themselves will be limited in their effectiveness.

So will prevention strategies that fail to take account of ''commonsense'' beliefs about health, illness and disease. It is often assumed that there is a direct link between knowledge and behaviour: once people are given the medical and scientific facts, they change their behaviour. Such simplistic assumptions are now known to be untrue. Everyday beliefs about diseases such as AIDS, which can distort the impact of health education messages, need to be taken into account — ''creatively'', says Dr Aggleton — in public information campaigns, peer education, and counselling.

Research is under way, in WHO and elsewhere, into the ways in which households and communities have responded to AIDS. Information from this work will shed light on how best to support affected families and communities. It may lead, too, to a clearer understanding of how to combat prejudice and discrimination against infected individuals and against groups popularly supposed to be at risk.

But social scientists frequently have to work in an atmosphere of suspicion and mistrust. Governments often fear that the information turned up by researchers may paint a less than favourable picture of how a society really operates. In some places, efforts have even been made to limit or forbid social and behavioural research. This is a challenge that has been taken up by WHO and others. If social scientists are allowed to carry out their research, the AIDS prevention activities they help design are bound to gain in effectiveness.

> In the face of the most deadly sexually transmitted disease ever to confront humanity, some would prohibit even the study of the human behaviors that put our children at risk. Thus we disarm ourselves in the middle of a lethal battle." — *US National Commission on AIDS (27)*

CHAPTER 18

Spreading the word about AIDS

There are no hard-to-reach people, only people who have not been reached.

Parked on a street busy with shoppers and office workers emerging into the warm evening air, Paisak Chom Muand waits for his taxi to fill with passengers before leaving for the city of Chiang Mai nestling in the mountains of northern Thailand. Paisak has been a taxi driver for 20 years, covering the route through the rice fields and small villages between San Sai and the city several times a day, carrying around a hundred passengers.

A couple of years back he heard that taxi drivers were invited to attend an AIDS information course at the local community hospital. "I didn't really believe then that AIDS existed," Paisak says. "I thought it was a government policy to eliminate brothels. But I went along anyway, and ended up as one of 14 drivers asked to become volunteer educators."

Since then, three of Paisak's regular passengers have died of AIDS. He has witnessed the distress of their families as mourners at the funerals have refused to touch the rice prepared, hurried away after the ceremony, and shunned them ever since. As a volunteer educator, with training and support from the health services, he gets regular supplies of AIDS information leaflets to tuck into the containers in his passenger cab, stickers with catchy messages about

AIDS, and condoms to offer to the passenger riding beside him if the opportunity should arise and the gesture seem appropriate.

Paisak says that practically all his passengers pick up a leaflet, and that today they are very ready to discuss AIDS as people they know begin to fall sick. An elderly relative in Paisak's own family recently died of AIDS. "No one wanted to touch him, or only with gloves on," he said. "But I knew from my training that there was nothing to fear and I should not keep away from him."

"Our assumption was that taxi drivers could be used very effectively as agents for change as they are in contact with so many people a day, and often ferry customers to the brothels," says Dr Surasing, a dentist in the office of the Provincial Medical Officer in Chiang Mai and the man behind the volunteer educator campaign. The team of around 80 taxi drivers in five districts is part of a larger campaign to reach out to people at the grass roots. Dr Surasing's network of volunteer educators includes hairdressers like Mrs Prathum, whose small, neat salon stands on a busy main road. She took up the work after frightened and ignorant people began whispering that having a haircut posed a danger of infection with HIV.

As she trims and curls and brushes, she engages her customers in conversation about AIDS, gently challenging denial, correcting misconceptions, and handing out leaflets they can take home. Mrs Prathum — married to a schoolteacher and mother of two daughters — feels a mission to protect people by passing on the knowledge she has gained about AIDS. Her salon has a reputation for rigorous hygiene and she proudly displays a notice in her window stating that she has passed her training with the health department and is one of their star educators.

Others in the network include brothel managers, prostitutes, Buddhist monks and "tuk-tuk" drivers, whose nippy, three-wheeled open vehicles are the most popular public transport in cities snarled with cars. Dr Surasing and his team have written a series of radio scripts.

Taxi driver Paisak Chom Muand, agent for change, hands out AIDS information to his passengers — and condoms too, if he feels the gesture is appropriate.

''No one listens when the government broadcasts information,'' he explains, ''so we pay popular disc jockeys to incorporate the messages we have scripted in their shows.'' The team also produces calendars for the general public — ''There's a different AIDS message on each page, and it has thirty days to sink in,'' says Dr Surasing — and videos for showing on the air-conditioned, long-haul buses running daily between Chiang Mai and Bangkok. These feature ordinary Thais who tell how they became infected with HIV, in an effort to dispel the belief that AIDS is always someone else's problem.

Evaluating the effectiveness of such an education campaign is extremely difficult, says Dr Surasing, but it is probably significant that the rate of new STD infections in Chiang Mai has slowed and that the incidence of HIV infection among sex workers appears to be stabilizing.

Central to the success of the campaign is the fact that it uses ''peer educators'' — people of the same background and social standing as their target audiences, who speak the same language, share the same values and know better than any outsider how to communicate with them. ''A major principle of good communication is to start from where people are, not where you think they are,'' says Dr Herbert Friedman, head of WHO's Adolescent Health Programme. ''This is much more difficult if education comes from professionals in ivory towers.'' It is a principle that has been widely recognized and applied in the fight against AIDS.

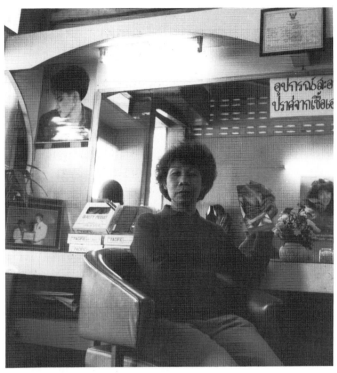

Hairdresser Mrs Prathum joined the network of community educators in Chiang Mai, Thailand, after people began to express fears that HIV could be transmitted during a haircut.

two weeks at lunch time and during free time between lessons. Teaching the basic facts about AIDS is the quickest and easiest part of the training. To give youngsters a deep appreciation of what AIDS means, and of the need for behaviour change, training also includes long discussion periods, role play (often based on newspaper cuttings collected by recruits), and meetings with people with AIDS. The peer

Youth to youth

Peer educators are used extensively in youth programmes. The assumption is that young people not only know best how to communicate with each other; they will also be trusted by their peers not to have a hidden agenda. Youngsters are often uniquely imaginative, using currently fashionable styles of music, theatre and art as powerful vehicles for information.

For example, Teens for AIDS Prevention (TAP), a project based in Washington, DC, recruits secondary school pupils to become peer educators, and gives them intensive training for

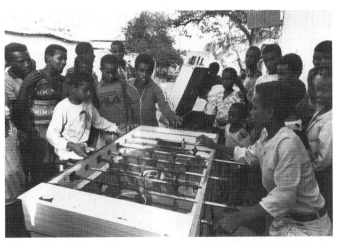

Sex and health education in schools will not reach the children who do not attend school. Special efforts are needed to make sure that all children get the information and skills they need to protect themselves from HIV.

educators then devise their own campaigns for use among their fellow students. One outcome has been a catchy song about AIDS called "Stupid Cupid".

However, the issue of teaching young people about sex and AIDS is often controversial. Many parents and school authorities fear that sex education will give approval — and even encouragement — to early sexual activity. "We adults deny adolescent sexuality hoping that if we don't think about it, it won't happen," says Dr Mariella Baldo, a youth expert in WHO's Global Programme on AIDS. "But there is a good deal of evidence that youngsters become sexually active far earlier than many adults are prepared to recognize." And there is now strong evidence from a number of surveys that sex education does *not* lead to early intercourse. If anything, it encourages responsibility: youngsters who have had sex education tend either to postpone intercourse or, if they do decide to have sex, use contraceptives.

"But we have learnt from experience that giving information is not enough on its own," says Dr Baldo. "If sex and AIDS education in schools is to be effective, young people must have access to condoms and to family planning and STD services. And they must learn the skills that are so crucial in sexual relationships.

"Giving young women decision-making and negotiating skills means, among other things, teaching them to recognize the consequences of their actions so that they can with-

draw from a potentially compromising situation before it goes too far," she explains.

Beyond the fringe

If peer education is useful with young people, it is even more crucial for groups of people who are stigmatized and harassed by mainstream society, and therefore suspicious of initiatives from outside.

One such group are sex workers, whose business is illegal in many countries, though often openly practised. An AIDS education campaign among female prostitutes in Accra, Ghana, began in 1987 with the training of six women who were articulate, had leadership qualities, and were respected by their fellow prostitutes (38). They worked with the project organizers to develop educational materials which they then distributed, along with free condoms and spermicide tablets, to their co-workers in Accra nightclubs. Each woman sought out ten of her colleagues to work with, informing them about the risks of HIV infection and encouraging them to use the condoms and/or spermicides.

The impact was remarkable. Before the project began only 13% of the prostitutes reported ever using condoms or spermicides. Three months into the project, a survey found that of 268 sexual contacts reported, 94% were protected by either condoms or spermicides or both. When the project was evaluated some months later, proportionately fewer of the women who had taken part tested positive for HIV than did prostitutes outside the project.

(More recent studies have sounded a word of warning about spermicides, which have been found to cause vaginal irritation — see Chapter 17.)

The AIDS Council of Southern Australia funded an effective peer group project organized by the Prostitutes Collective of Victoria, Melbourne. The female sex workers involved in the project, whose trade had been driven underground by oppressive laws and police action, had been considered particularly hard to reach through other strategies (39). A dynamic peer educator, trained by a health centre and the Family Planning Association, contacted many prostitutes working secretly from home, giving them information and ad-

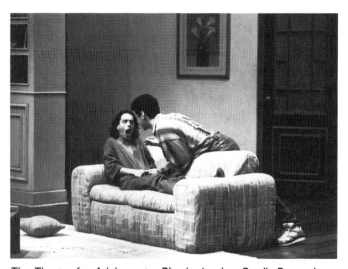

The Theatre for Adolescents, Rio de Janeiro, Brazil. Drama is an excellent vehicle for information about AIDS. It holds the audience's attention and is an acceptable way of bringing up sensitive or taboo issues that people find hard to talk about in other settings.

vice about HIV/AIDS, and low-cost condoms. The Collective also published a bimonthly newsletter called *Working Girl*, with articles written by prostitutes about many aspects of their work, including those related to AIDS, STD, and prevention of violence. The Collective has also been involved in negotiations with the government on changes in the law.

In Ethiopia in 1989, a nurse-counsellor called Aster Wolde Kidane started a peer education project in Addis Ababa after a serosurvey revealed that many of the city's sex workers were HIV-positive. She encouraged a group of women working at the poorest end of the sex trade, operating out of their own tiny, backstreet rooms, to organize themselves into a mutual support group.

Supervising weekly meetings in a room behind the local community clinic, Sister Aster trained the literate women to teach the others about AIDS using colourful pictorial flip charts to stimulate discussion. The meetings have become a springboard for other activities, too. The group has started saving money in the hope of eventually starting their own café or handicraft stall. Each week there are women spinning cotton, deftly rolling the spindle along their thighs, as one of their colleagues leads the discussion on AIDS and hands out condom supplies.

According to the women, the main benefit they derive from the group is the feeling of control and the enhanced self-respect it gives them. Almaz, for example, felt very frightened and helpless when she first heard about AIDS over the grapevine. But now, she says, she has the knowledge and the means to protect herself, and finds little resistance from clients to condom use because everyone is becoming aware. "Before when we got sick there was no one to care. Now we try to look after our health, and we look after each other. Sister Aster is a real friend to us, and the group is like having a family."

Some projects have effectively used non-peer educators to reach people living on the fringes of society. In the *Pegação* project in Rio de Janeiro, Brazil, a team composed mainly of young psychologists provides education, counselling and condoms to young male prostitutes, mostly aged between 11 and 23 years, who hang out in the Copacabana area looking for clients. *Pegação*, which is a slang expression meaning "to cruise", started in 1989 after a survey revealed that 43% of the male prostitutes tested were HIV-positive.

Comprehensive prevention: what will it cost?

Even in the absence of a vaccine, further spread of HIV is not inevitable. People can be convinced and helped to avoid risky behaviour, by means of information through the mass media, educational programmes, condom promotion, and other methods of proven effectiveness. Where prevention has been approached in this way, the results have been remarkably successful. But, except in a handful of countries, these tried and tested approaches have not been applied widely enough to make a real impact on the epidemic.

One reason is that prevention programmes have been starved of resources. Only an estimated US$ 120 million was spent on AIDS prevention in the entire developing world in 1992 — ten to twenty times too little. According to research carried out by WHO, annual expenditure on prevention will have to be increased to between $1500 million and $2900 million in order to make a significant difference to the rate of new infections in developing countries. This is what it would cost to get a "basic prevention package" operating in all developing countries.

The project team first visited the areas where the young men operate and talked to them about their lives and concerns. "[We found that] to survive was much more important [to them] than to live well or to have any kind of personal care", says Paulo Henrique Longo, *Pegação*'s coordinator. AIDS was not a priority; their lives were already plagued by hunger, fear and violence. Because many did not consider themselves homosexual and indeed had wives or girlfriends (who knew nothing of their activity), they did not consider AIDS messages addressed to homosexuals to have anything to do with them. Many could not even understand the written materials because they were illiterate, while others were reluctant to carry leaflets for fear of police harassment or arrest.

The team realized that most of the young men were isolated and had low self-esteem. The first task was therefore to win their trust by being regularly available and showing concern for all their problems; only then would they be receptive to AIDS information. Team members have become familiar faces in the area. They hold regular meetings at bars and cafés in town where discussion is encouraged and safer sex practices are explored through games. The team

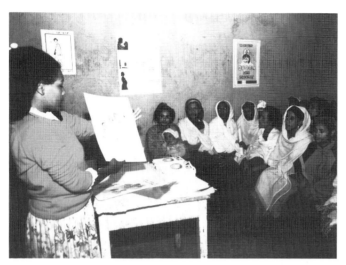

With encouragement from Sister Aster Wolde — a nurse-counsellor — sex workers in Addis Ababa who are normally isolated in their work have formed a support group. They meet to exchange information, learn about HIV/AIDS, distribute condoms, and support each other in pressing clients to use them.

also works with the young men to create AIDS information materials that are relevant to their lives. The objective is to build self-esteem at the same time as creating awareness. "It is important to listen to the men rather than to talk at them," said Mr Longo, "because the factors that induce behaviour change are different with each individual."

Pegação's results have been impressive. Within six months of its starting, the proportion of young men attached to the project who reported that they always used condoms increased from 15% to 65% — a figure which had gone up to 80% by the end of the first year. The proportion who reported never using condoms fell from 77% to 7%. Tellingly, the great majority of newcomers are introduced to the programme by other male prostitutes who have already benefited (40). *Pegação* has been elected to represent community-based organizations on the State Commission which is responsible for AIDS policy in Rio de Janeiro.

However, the project has had little success in one area — improving the men's access to health care. This is in part because of laws that require minors to have an adult authorize their treatment, and in part because of the reluctance of health workers to treat prostitutes.

A programme similar to *Pegação* operates among men who have sex with men in Australia. Called the "Sydney Beats Outreach Project", it makes contact with men in the Sydney area who are not part of the organized gay community, by going to the places where they seek out sex partners. Known as "beats", these include beaches, public toilets and parks, and roadside rest-stops. The project was developed because of sociological research which revealed that although considerable behaviour change had occurred within organized gay communities, largely through community-level efforts, there were many homosexually active men who were not being reached by any of these interventions because of their social and geographical isolation (41).

In Scotland, a gay "outreach" project run by Scottish AIDS Monitor (SAM) takes AIDS information and safer sex messages to the places in Edinburgh and Glasgow where homosexually active men meet. "We have a problem here in that some of the younger men entering the gay scene see AIDS as an 'older man's problem' that doesn't really concern them," says Paul Trainer of SAM. Furthermore, he says, male prostitution is on the increase in Scotland's large cities, much of it related to maintaining a drug or alcohol habit, and the incidence of violence against homosexuals, directly related to the commercial sex scene, is rising. "However, because of AIDS, these controversial issues like poverty, drug use, sexuality, which had been successfully swept under the carpet, are being looked at again and debated."

Besides seeking out their target audience in the popular cruising spots and bars, SAM's workers try to cast their net more widely with their "Safer Sex Roadshow".

Bombay Dost, founded in 1990, was one of the first gay organizations in India, where homosexuality is heavily stigmatized. The organization's goal is to provide a forum in which gay men and lesbians can explore what it means to be homosexual in India, and to advocate the legal and social acceptance of homosexuality. Among its projects are safer-sex workshops, counselling, and the publication of a magazine, *Bombay Dost,* with articles on a wide range of issues of special concern to its readers, including information about gay organizations in other Indian states and abroad.

Issues of credibility

The credibility of the "messenger" is all-important in AIDS awareness campaigns, and people with personal experience of HIV infection or AIDS are some of the most believable messengers around. "PWAs [people with AIDS] have crossed a certain threshold. They already have the disease which scares everyone half to death. They've had to learn to live with that fear and many of them have transcended it. We can help people to learn to overcome the fear which blinds them to realities of AIDS," said Richard Rector, a member of WHO's Advisory Council on AIDS (*42*).

Rector is one of a growing number of people with AIDS in many countries who are active in the campaign to halt the epidemic. Besides lending their hard-earned expertise to the planning of campaigns and creation of educational material, many go in person to address groups in factories, colleges, schools. By so doing they give a human face to the facts and figures, and substance to the threat, which helps break down the belief that "AIDS could never happen to me".

Their invaluable contribution has been recognized by the Secretary-General of the United Nations, Dr Boutros Boutros-Ghali, who paid special tribute to people with AIDS during an address to the United Nations General Assembly in New York in 1992. Appealing to others to speak out, Dr Boutros-Ghali said: "It

A PWA tells his story

Donald de Gagné, a former radio producer with the Canadian Broadcasting Corporation, was diagnosed with AIDS on his 31st birthday, in January 1988. Doctors gave him only months to live. Almost six years later, he campaigns internationally for people with AIDS (PWAs), working at a pace that would tax anyone. Since 1989 he has been director of the Vancouver PWA Society, addressing issues such as clinical trials, policy-making, human rights, and the role of PWAs in health care.

"[Being diagnosed with AIDS was] a major shock, because when you are young you never think about dying. You feel you are almost invincible. You are thinking about the future, your career, about changing the world and having a relationship. And then suddenly somebody puts a spoke in the wheel. In one day you go through many different feelings — isolation, fear, a feeling that your life is going to end very soon — and you cry a lot to let go of things that you believed were going to happen. Crying is OK. You have to go through that phase. But you get sick and tired of it after a while and you just have to pick up your courage and deal with what is coming.

"When you live with AIDS for a long time — and I feel I am breaking ground in this area — you can burn out. You lose a lot of friends and everything is changing around you. I think that is the hardest thing about AIDS: to learn how to grow with the changes all the time. Your health is changing, the people around you are changing, the disease itself is changing. All your terms of reference are constantly being put to the test and you have to reorientate yourself constantly."

As a member of an international network of PWAs, de Gagné visited Rwanda in 1992 to help people with AIDS in Kigali to develop their own support group. "When I arrived, absolutely nobody with AIDS was visible. I had a list of about a dozen people who had agreed to talk to me. They had been told I had AIDS, and I talked to them individually. I was just amazed and very touched by how they opened up to me and trusted me.

"The key word that came out was isolation. They were just so isolated. They had nobody to talk to and felt so desperate. So seven of the people I met volunteered to be founding organizers, and we had a founding meeting on the evening I had to catch my plane."

Persuading society at large that people with AIDS should be included in the campaign against the epidemic is a constant uphill struggle, says de Gagné. "Quite frankly, people with AIDS are easily discarded. Many people believe they are not worth investing in even in terms of treatment or access to health care, or in terms of money for an air ticket [to attend an international conference]. But for us everybody is a human being and should be respected as that."

is thanks to them, thanks to their open words that the authorities in the communities where they live will take initiatives. And these initiatives will be of benefit not only to the community of the sick; it will also be very useful as a means of prevention.''

Given the level of discrimination against them, it takes commitment, vision and tremendous courage for people with HIV infection or AIDS to reveal their condition. However, the benefit flows both ways: for such individuals to be active campaigners rather than passive recipients of care, pity and prejudice is life-affirming and, some believe, helps to keep physical illness at bay. ''When you have AIDS so much is taken from you. But speaking to young people gives me back something,'' said Paul Maignot from Toronto, Canada (43). ''I'm not a person with AIDS waiting to die. I'm a person fighting for my life, fighting for understanding and fighting to educate others that yes, this *could* happen to them.''

Robert Mugemana, a Rwandan and one of the first people with AIDS in Africa to commit himself openly to AIDS prevention, said: ''I had no one to talk to, no shoulder to lean on when I was struck with HIV. I don't want anyone to go through that nightmare. This is the only way I can hit back at the disease which turned my entire life upside down'' (42). Mugemana died in 1992.

In the war against ignorance, imagination is the key to reaching people. However, creating awareness is insufficient in itself to stop the spread of the virus, for long experience has taught that there is no direct connection between knowledge and behaviour change. As the following chapters will show, information and education are just one part of an interdependent package of preventive measures that are truly effective only if applied together.

CHAPTER 19

New rules for an old game: promoting safer sex

"Protecting yourself from AIDS is not something you can do on your own. It takes the mutual support of both partners. And that in turn is possible only when the preventive behaviour is valued by the social group you belong to." — Daniel Defert, France (44)

The rules of the game have changed with the advent of AIDS. Communities are under threat from long-standing practices which have suddenly become deadly, such as unprotected casual sex.

But encouraging safer sexual practices means negotiating a path through the minefield of taboos, prejudices and inhibitions that surround sexual activity in almost every society — a task made more difficult by the problems associated with the condom, at present the only mechanical barrier to the sexual transmission of HIV.

The male condom has a long history both as a contraceptive and as a barrier against disease. Ancient Egyptians used sheaths of animal membrane to prevent pregnancy, and in 16th-century Italy the anatomist Fallopius designed a linen sheath to protect against syphilis. The device itself is said to derive its name from a Dr Condom who made sheaths for King Charles II of England in the 17th century.

Today, in the absence of either a vaccine or cure, latex condoms have a vital role in the fight against AIDS. It is important to give people the full range of options for preventing sexual transmission: abstinence, mutual fidelity, non-penetrative sex, and intercourse protected by a condom. The experience of national AIDS programmes during the past ten years shows that condom use is often the method selected.

Unfortunately, condoms have a serious image problem. In many parts of the world,

they are widely associated with prostitution, casual affairs, and STD prevention. People say condoms reduce intimacy and impair sensation. For example, sex with a condom has been compared to eating a sweet with the wrapper on.

In developed countries, the sheath's popularity fell sharply with the advent of the contraceptive pill and intrauterine device (IUD). Except in Japan, where 45% of all couples — 69% of family planning users — rely on condoms, their use by married couples in the developed world has fallen to between 5% and 15%. In developing countries, only 4% of married couples use condoms, and in sub-Saharan Africa the figure is often below 1%.

There are also cultural obstacles to the condom's use. "In sub-Saharan Africa, we have an expression: skin to skin", says Dr Faustin Yao of GPA's Youth and General Public unit. "A condom interferes with the traditional 'mystical' meaning of sexual intercourse because it blocks skin contact and prevents the man's sperm from being deposited in the woman. Interestingly", he adds, "women seem more prepared than men to forego this contact and use a condom if it means avoiding a fatal disease — perhaps because they are the ones who care for the sick and dying, and death for them is more vivid, more real."

Technical problems serve to undermine confidence further. In many countries people say that condoms tear — especially those bought from open-air markets, where they have been exposed to sunlight, tropical humidity and pollution. The risk of damage to a condom is greater in anal intercourse than in vaginal or oral sex. And when condoms are used as contraceptives they have a failure rate of about 12% in the first year, before couples become experienced. It must be stressed, however, that the effectiveness of a condom depends on how consistently it is used: *the most common reason for its failure as a contraceptive is the couple's failure to use it every time they have intercourse.*

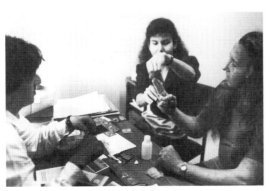

A doctor in São Paulo, Brazil, explains to a male sex worker how condoms should be used.

In many countries, family planning associations have taken up the challenge of improving the condom's image, promoting it as a device that has no side-effects, is safe for young people to use, and requires no medical supervision. In Colombia, the Profamilia organization managed to increase condom sales by 50% through an intensive advertising campaign. Elsewhere, too, family planning associations have established imaginative programmes to promote condoms. Some have set aside ''male hours'' at their clinics; some have set up AIDS telephone hotlines (particularly popular with young people); and some have launched special projects catering for the counselling and condom needs of men who have sex with men (45).

Some, like the Planned Parenthood Association of Ghana, collaborate with trade-unions and business management to provide regular training sessions and distribute condoms in the workplace. The Association has also established special clubs for men in some rural areas. The clubs are primarily recreational, but they use the regular evening gatherings to discuss health and sex and to provide condoms. They also encourage fathers to talk to their sons about sex and advise them on how to approach the subject (46).

However, it would be a mistake to put the responsibility for condom promotion on family planning programmes alone. Some family planning staff are reluctant to take on AIDS work, or worry that the association with disease might affect the image of family planning. In any case, family planning programmes could not possibly integrate AIDS prevention into their normal work without extra staff, specialist training, transport, equipment and outreach.

Condoms as a commodity

One particularly effective way of getting condoms to those who need them is through ''social marketing'': the application of commercial sales and marketing techniques to a public health problem. ''Using the private sector and its distribution networks makes condoms readily available to people in ways that public health programmes usually cannot,'' explained Carlos Ferreros, who has directed condom social marketing programmes in a number of countries. ''You can buy Coca-Cola, beer, cigarettes just about anywhere. No matter how bad the roads are, no matter how rural the village, there's always some villager getting goods out there'' (47).

Successful social marketing depends on having the right product at the right price in the right place, backed up by the right promotion. It has been used for decades to promote family planning, oral rehydration for diarrhoea, STD treatment and other public health goals. Since the advent of AIDS, social marketing has moved condoms into some of the remotest corners of the world, particularly in Africa. In Zaire, whose 35 million people are widely scattered across a land with very poor communications, condom distribution soared from less than half a million in 1987 to 8 million in 1990 and 18 million in 1991 (40) as a small army of salesmen working on commission took boats, trains, trucks, and, where necessary, walked to reach remote villages with their product.

In Ethiopia, condoms used to be distributed almost exclusively through family planning clinics, which served married couples only. Condoms were one of the least popular methods of contraception: in 1987, only about 20 000 were distributed nationwide. But in 1991, just one year after Ethiopia's social marketing

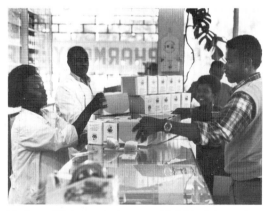

Teshome Wakene, a salesman with Ethiopia's condom social marketing programme, distributes condoms through all kinds of commercial outlets, from pharmacies to street kiosks, from bars to petrol stations. Wakene and his colleagues have been so successful in overcoming public reluctance to discuss or use condoms that the programme has trouble keeping up with demand.

programme was launched, sales of condoms shot up to 6 million. Despite logistic problems caused by the civil war, condoms were available in around 100 towns and villages. And soldiers from the army of Mengistu Haile Mariam, the former Ethiopian ruler, received a take-home pack of AIDS information and condoms on demobilization.

"A couple of years ago, you couldn't mention the word condom," says Teshome Wakene, an enthusiastic young sales representative with Population Services International (PSI-Ethiopia), which runs the country's social marketing programme. "At first, people were shy about asking for them at street kiosks, pharmacies and such places. But I tell them that condoms are just like medicines; they protect us from disease and save our lives, and no one would be shy about asking for medicine if they needed it. Now everyone talks about them."

Teshome spends most of his working day on the road, doing the rounds of small shops, bars, hotels and even petrol stations, which he has identified as good places to reach the long-distance lorry drivers whose way of life makes them particularly vulnerable to HIV infection. Along the narrow streets of the *mercato* — one of the biggest and busiest markets in Africa — he ducks into the tiny rooms of prostitutes. With friendly greetings, he opens his blue suitcase to hand out packets of "Hiwot" condoms, (the word means "life" in Amharic), AIDS information material, and a key-ring/condom holder with the Hiwot logo, as a free gift for his customer.

Teshome and his fellow sales representatives sell the condoms at 25 US cents for a packet of four, and their customers re-sell them for 30 cents. The small profit made by the retailers gives them an incentive to stock the product.

One of Teshome's best customers is Mrs Askala Tekale, proprietor of the Blue Nile Bar in a square in central Addis Ababa. A large, friendly woman, she sits in the bar's backyard under a washing-line of lacy underwear and tells why she is so committed to condoms. As a housewife, she bought the bar in the early 1980s to make some extra money. But, she chuckles, selling beer without sex is not very profitable, so she engaged a number of young women to sell drinks and began renting out rooms behind the bar to customers. When she found that pregnancy among the bar-girls was a big problem, she started promoting condoms.

"Mrs Tekale already had stickers on her walls saying 'no sex without condoms' when we first came to discuss our selling campaign with her," says Teshome. Today she talks about AIDS with her customers, who are mostly teachers, students and office workers. She has put Hiwot dispensers beside the bar and in the public toilets and says that resistance to their use has all but vanished as awareness of the epidemic has grown.

PSI-Ethiopia also has a high-school programme. Operating through the various special-interest students' clubs, it reaches around 120 000 young people in 27 schools with AIDS information and condoms. A student representative at each school takes delivery of condoms from PSI and pays the programme back from the proceeds of previous sales. According to Zenebework Bissrat, the programme officer, at first there was resistance to the idea of giving AIDS information in schools, as parents and education authorities chose to ignore the evidence that young unmarried people are sexually active. "Virginity is much prized," she says, "and adults were blinding themselves to the fact that teenage pregnancy is on the increase in Ethiopia and youngsters are contracting HIV."

The job of PSI-Ethiopia's salesforce is helped greatly by the national AIDS programme, whose imaginative "Fight AIDS Together" campaign trains representatives from a whole range of grass-roots organizations — from community and church groups to profes-

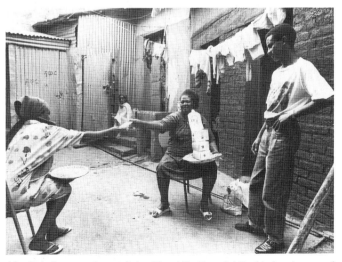

Mrs Tekale, proprietor of the Blue Nile Bar, Addis Ababa, is one of the condom social marketing programme's best customers. She is strongly committed to the use of condoms on her premises.

sional associations and government departments — to act as peer educators. The information campaign also uses mass media and popular culture such as drama, songs and poetry to educate and inform. The result is high levels of awareness about HIV/AIDS, especially in urban areas, and high demand for condoms. The national AIDS programme has also organized campaigns targeted at sex workers in some of the busier towns.

The main problem for Ethiopia's social marketing programme has been keeping up with condom demand and ensuring continued supplies to customers even when political instability disrupts the marketing network. In the busy market town of Nazareth, an effective peer education and condom supply programme for sex workers almost collapsed in late 1991 when civil war reached the town, community health posts were destroyed and looted of equipment, and peer educators fled home to their villages.

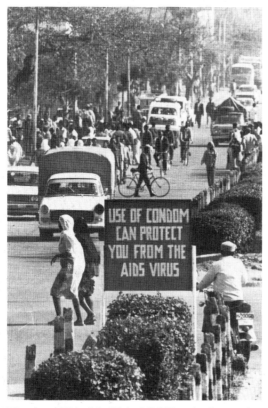

The aim of Ethiopia's "Fight AIDS Together" campaign is to spread information as widely as possible about HIV and how to prevent infection. This road sign is in Nazareth.

Targeting the most vulnerable

Constrained by lack of money, bad roads, lack of transport, and short supplies, some countries concentrate their efforts on condom promotion among people thought to be most vulnerable to HIV infection, rather than try to cover the whole population. One such country is the United Republic of Tanzania where, in September 1989, the African Medical and Research Foundation (AMREF) started a project focusing on long-distance truckers and their sex partners.

The job of Christopher Mwaijonga, a Health and Behaviour Officer with AMREF, is to visit the truck stops along the busy highways connecting the Tanzanian capital, Dar es Salaam, to neighbouring countries. Many truck stops have become satellite communities by drawing people from remote villages to trade, catch transport, or offer services to the passing traffic. Truck drivers and their crews spend their leisure hours here relaxing in the myriad brightly lit bars and small hotels with such names as "The Just Imagine Hotel", "The Paris Centre" and the "Welcome Good Time Shop". Drink, companionship and casual sex are abundantly on offer.

"We had some opposition at first from church leaders who thought promoting condoms would also promote promiscuity," says Mwaijonga. "But I told them the time would come when priests would face only empty benches on Sundays if we didn't recognize reality and take the steps necessary to control the spread of HIV."

Mwaijonga is responsible for recruiting candidates from among the bar girls and bar owners to be trained as peer educators, and for supervising and supporting them after training. To be effective, candidates must have the approval and support not just of their co-workers, but of hotel proprietors and local community leaders also. And, once trained, they need recognition as valued and expert members of the AMREF team, for their job is tough and stressful. "Some of the girls I work with are very resistant to my messages," says Siasa, leaning against a bar stool in the sticky heat of a Tanzanian summer night. "Their attitude is that they know me well, they grew up with me, and what can I teach them?" But Siasa, one of the most committed of the project's 20 peer educators, knows her colleagues take in what she says about AIDS because she has seen the demand for condoms rise steadily.

When women go into bars to talk about AIDS they sometimes meet with intense hostility, even violence, from truckers, who resent being singled out by the AIDS campaign. "I don't think we have done enough to avoid discrimination against truckers," says Dr Ulrich Laukamm-Josten, Director of AMREF in the United Republic of Tanzania. "We have talked a lot about the role truckers have played in spreading HIV infection in Africa without due regard to their sensibilities. The life of a trucker is full of frustrations, and at night they stop and drink and have sex as a way of compensating for all this. They are understandably hostile if they think someone has stigmatized their way of life and is trying to interfere with it."

But over the years, the kindly, non-judgemental manner of Christopher Mwaijonga and his colleagues has earned respect and softened resistance. Many of the trucks have AIDS and condom stickers displayed on cabin windows. And today, education sessions in the bars are often crowded, lively occasions for discussion and questioning. "We have a rule that educators mustn't give just any answer to a query. If they don't know something they must say so, and tell the enquirer they'll find out," says Mwaijonga.

Distribution of condoms at the truck stops rose from 60 000 between September and December 1989 to almost 700 000 between January and April 1991. Moreover, the proportion of women at the truck stops who reported using condoms increased from 50% to 90% over the 16-month period to mid-1991. For men, the reported increase was from 54% to 74% (40). Guest house proprietors report greater demand for condoms and say that truckers sometimes ask about the availability of condoms before booking a room (48).

Laukamm-Josten believes the project will have an effect far beyond the highway out of Dar Es Salaam. "When truckers go back to their village, they take along new ideas. If they've been using condoms they'll take some back home and word will get around that they're using such things. This will have a profound effect on their peers," he says. "Eventually they'll run out of condoms and not be able to

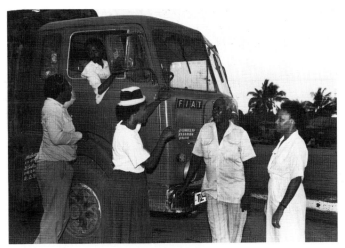

AMREF field workers talk to drivers at a truck stop on a main road as part of their AIDS information and condom promotion campaign.

get any at the village store. So, because they know that unprotected sex is dangerous, they will reduce their sexual activity for a while until they can get more supplies or leave again for work. Gradually a pattern of using condoms or saying 'no' to sex will become established. We have no proof that this is happening, but a lot of anecdotal evidence. This is the kind of behaviour change that is going to be necessary to stop the epidemic."

An evaluation of AMREF's truckers project found that many of the women were reportedly unable to insist on condom use with reluctant customers, some of whom offer extra

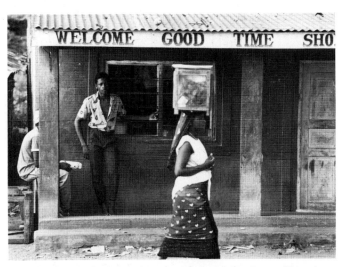

Truck stops on a busy highway are places of transience. Many have become satellite communities as people from isolated villages come to the roadside to trade, catch transport, or offer services to the passing traffic. These provide fertile conditions for the spread of HIV.

money or threaten violence to get unprotected sex (48). This is a common and worldwide problem that consistently undermines the effort to contain AIDS. AMREF is considering special training to help the women stand up for themselves.

Redressing the balance of power

At a massage parlour in an Asian resort, a woman in a short dress and fishnet tights stands up and turns to face her colleagues who sit in a pool of light on the dance-floor combing their hair, appraising their make-up with tiny hand-mirrors, or laughing softly with their friends. Sex Worker Number 236, according to a card pinned to her dress, she is about to demonstrate how to open a condom packet with long finger-nails without tearing it, and how to put it on a customer in a pleasurable way. She tilts her head and giggles at the peal of laughter from the floor as she strokes the condom onto an outstretched finger with exaggerated movements.

But the lesson being taught to the young women on the dance-floor is being undermined by the bar owner, who sits watching the demonstration with a small group of customers. "What goes on between the girl and the customer is their own business," she says. "The management doesn't insist on condoms or interfere with the transaction even if a customer gets rough with a girl. There's too much competition in this town."

It was to change working practices like these, and to create an environment supportive of safer sex, that Thailand's national AIDS programme conceived the "100% condom campaign". The principle is that all sex establishments in an area should adopt a "no sex without a condom" policy simultaneously, so that customers cannot threaten to go to the brothel next door to avoid condoms (40).

The campaign is administered by local governments, which are responsible for convincing the owners of all sex establishments in their area of the AIDS threat and explaining the scheme. Brothel owners are told that the women will be checked regularly for STDs, and that there will be penalties, ranging from fines to

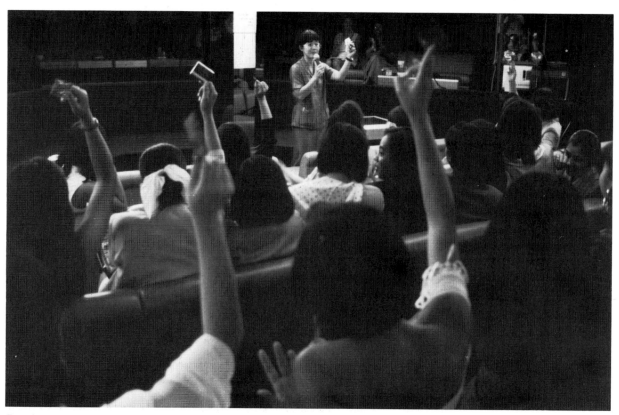

Female sex workers at a massage parlour watch a condom demonstration.

closure of the premises, for non-compliance with the condom rule. In addition to the prostitutes and their clients, key players in the campaign are the health sector, which provides STD services, health education and condoms, and is responsible for monitoring the incidence of STDs; and the police, who act on information from STD clinics to penalize establishments whose workers continue to contract such diseases — evidence that condom use is less than 100%.

Brothel owners also have an interest in keeping to the rules, says Dr Surasing, an enthusiastic advocate of the campaign. "Having several of your girls off work because of STDs costs money and gives the brothel a bad name. Those kinds of problems are avoided if condoms are always used."

The campaign has had its problems. Initially, for example, too little effort was made to inform the sex workers about the campaign, or to involve them in decisions about how to implement it — both of which would have ensured better cooperation from these key players.

After some of these problems were resolved, the campaign was expanded and by early 1992 it was operating in 66 of Thailand's 73 provinces. Surveys to assess its effectiveness have found that STD prevalence has declined spectacularly, from 13% to less than 0.5% among sex workers in Samut Sakhon, for example, where the number of condoms distributed in brothels increased almost fourfold within a month of the campaign's introduction. In Chiang Mai, Thailand's northern province which has been particularly badly affected by AIDS, condom use among sex workers is reported to have increased by 50 – 60% since the start of the campaign.

Thailand's "100% condom campaign" has been an initiative from the top. "In many countries, the first to recognize the need for condom use and to take decisive steps to empower women have been women themselves," says Priscilla Alexander, an expert on prostitution. In countries as diverse as Australia, Ethiopia, and the Philippines, to name just a few, sex workers have formed collectives based on mutual support, and adopted community-based policies whereby condoms are compulsory and customers who resist are not served. Such organi-

zations also give heavily stigmatized and marginalized sex workers a way to voice their concerns and press for their rights — notably an end to oppressive laws and law enforcement practices. Such laws drive prostitution underground and thereby make every aspect of HIV/AIDS prevention more difficult — from holding educational gatherings, to creating information materials targeted at sex workers, to carrying condoms. For example, if Mrs Tekale or the sex workers of Ethiopia's *mercato* feared arrest or prosecution, they would not be so willing to cooperate with PSI's social marketing campaign, which draws attention to their activities.

Often the most successful "safer sex" projects among prostitutes are those that do not focus just on AIDS but also concern themselves with the other problems of their daily lives, such as discrimination against their children, police harassment and violence by clients.

"It is essential for funding bodies and educators alike to understand that AIDS cannot be treated as a single and separate issue in the sex industry," says Andi Sebastian of the Prostitutes Collective of Victoria. "AIDS is one risk in a series of risks. It is one reason to be terrified amongst many reasons to be ter-

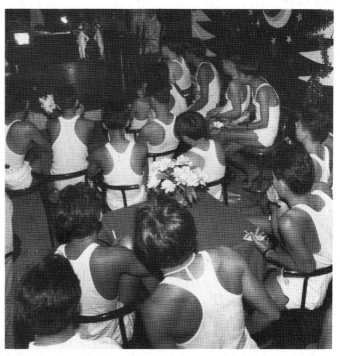

Male sex workers in Pattaya, Thailand, receive information about AIDS and safer sex from an outreach team sent by the local STD clinic.

rified. It is one problem to deal with amongst many. AIDS is an occupational health and safety issue, it is an economic factor, it is a personal concern and it is one of an infinite variety of factors which marginalise sex workers in the community'' (*39*).

This is a message that holds true beyond the world of commercial sex, too. Unless AIDS prevention projects are based on a full understanding of the reality of people's lives and the driving forces behind their behaviour, they have little chance of success.

CHAPTER 20

Beating prejudice: AIDS prevention among drug injectors

"Many people like to think that [injecting] drug use is not their problem, since they have nothing to do with junkies. But they would be surprised to see the make-up of people in our treatment programs. The addict is your doctor, your police officer, your bus driver. Many people go to work every day and nobody knows about their addiction. They carry this secret with them, and the fear that someone will find out about it." — *Yolanda Serrano, USA (49)*

The effort to control the spread of HIV among people who inject drugs is greatly complicated by the fact that the taking of drugs, other than tobacco and (in most countries) alcohol, is almost universally condemned. In many countries, harsh laws and diligent policing drive drug users beyond the reach of health and social services into a twilight world of secrecy and fear, largely ignored by the rest of society.

AIDS brought a new urgency to the debate about how best to deal with drugs, highlighting the age-old controversies and moral dilemmas surrounding this issue. But, says Jo Kittelsen, a Norwegian specialist in programmes for injecting drug users, "the good news is that drug injectors are able and willing to change their practices to reduce the risk of HIV infections if they get the right support."

Today, more than a decade into the epidemic, there is solid evidence that several different approaches work, all of them based on a non-judgemental attitude towards drug users and practical support to help them avoid getting infected with HIV through contaminated injection equipment. For example, programmes for the distribution of clean needles and syringes have been used successfully in many countries including Australia, Canada, the Netherlands, New Zealand, Sweden, and the United Kingdom; while bleach distribution is more popular in places where needles and syringes are too costly to give away.

There has been strong political opposition to these harm-reduction programmes in many countries on the grounds that they send the "wrong message" to drug users and undermine the war on drugs. However, the police often tolerate unofficial syringe exchanges, such as those in Tacoma, Washington, and San Francisco in the USA. Most important, the evidence refutes the claim that such programmes result in increased drug use. In Amsterdam, for example, neither the total number of drug injec-

tors, nor the frequency with which individuals inject, has increased since syringe exchanges were opened (*50*).

The first syringe exchange in the United Kingdom was established in 1986. Since 1987, when the government gave its approval of the strategy, more than 200 syringe exchanges have opened. A triumph of pragmatism over prejudice, the exchanges have become the cornerstone of the effort to control the spread of HIV among injecting drug users in Britain (*64*). The fact is that AIDS is a deadlier threat than drug use. Exchanges do not condone the use of drugs, says Gerry Stimson, Director of the London-based Centre for Research on Drugs and Health Behaviour, but they recognize the need to work with people who continue to inject drugs in order to reduce HIV transmission.

Syringe exchanges are not always readily accepted by the local community, however, so they need to be carefully planned and tailored to meet the needs of both the target audiences and the neighbourhoods in which they live.

Trial and error bring success in Glasgow

"Our first attempt at operating a syringe exchange was not a success," says John Cameron, coordinator of Glasgow's programme. "The place was picketed for six months by local residents who claimed that crime would increase, that their streets would be littered with used needles, and that people would be dealing and injecting outside. Consequently, injecting drug users were a rare species at that first exchange."

After 18 months, the project was still seeing only 15 to 25 people a week out of a drug injecting population estimated at between 8 000 and 12 000. One mistake was that the syringe exchange was housed in an unattractive building that afforded very little privacy to visitors because it was exposed; furthermore, it was inaccessible to many parts of the city. So the first place was closed and the programme moved to the heart of the communities where it was most needed. There, it achieved swift success. Within three months of opening its doors, one exchange had more than 150 clients, most of whom were local people who used it regularly. Moreover, it had a return rate of used equipment of more than 100% as clients started bringing in for safe disposal syringes they had bought at pharmacies (51).

By the end of 1991 there were six syringe exchanges in Glasgow, with others planned. The number of attendances at the exchanges that year was around 21 000, during which some 190 000 syringes were handed out, with a return rate of 130%.

"It's essential to prepare the ground care-

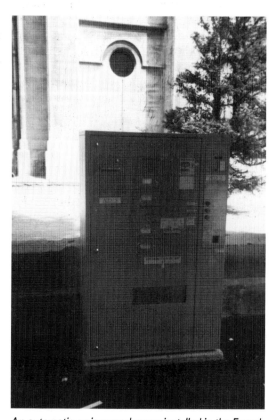

An automatic syringe exchanger installed in the French city of Nîmes in July 1993 with the help of AIDES, one of France's first AIDS self-help associations. In exchange for their old syringe and needle, clients get a kit comprising two new syringes, disinfectant, condoms, and information about services available for clients wishing to stop drug use.

fully before starting a project," says John Cameron. "I start by visiting and talking to everyone, from members of parliament and the local council to the community groups." Gaining the confidence of the community is particularly important, he says, because drug injectors naturally fear that such a project will expose them to the police (drug use is illegal) or to social workers, who might evict them from their homes.

One of Britain's earliest exchanges opened in Easterhouse, a grey high-rise estate sandwiched between motorways on the outskirts of Glasgow, where groups of unemployed young people stand on exposed street corners. "The drug problem here is all tied up with hopelessness and helplessness. Half the people on this estate have no jobs," said John Cameron, leaning against a table in the brightly lit community exchange one April evening, while a steady stream of clients passed through.

Opening plastic carrier bags before the health worker seated at a big table, clients showed what used equipment they had brought back before dropping the package into the big bin. They discussed with the worker what kind of clean needles they wanted to take away, how many condoms, and whether they wanted bleach to clean their needles in an emergency. And for those with health or other worries, there were specialist staff — including a community nurse and psychiatric nurses — available down the hall.

"My view is that the problem exists, you can't ignore it, and it's my duty to try to prevent people harming themselves," said a nurse who has unique insight into the community in which she works because she grew up there herself. "One lad I saw tonight had an abscess and a mottled leg he was in danger of losing. But some people just like to have someone taking care of them and showing them respect."

John — a thin, nervous, blond-haired man in his late twenties who said he had been injecting drugs for 10 years — came in with two friends. The three were enthusiastic clients of the exchange. "Before this place opened life was really dangerous," said John. "You couldn't get the kind of equipment you wanted, so you used to share, and to use a needle until it was like an old nail and your veins collapsed." He shook his head at the memory. "Now I can get new needles and special plastic containers that keep them safely out of the reach of my kids."

Like John, many drug users are family people, and the fear that their children will be taken away is one of the things that keeps them away from drug programmes.

At Easterhouse there is a security guard at the door to ensure that no drug dealing goes on nearby — a situation which would undermine public support for the project — and clients are not permitted to inject on the premises. "We took these decisions because we can't be responsible for clients harming themselves or overdosing. You learn what rules are necessary as you go along," says Cameron.

How effective are syringe exchanges?

Syringe exchanges in the United Kingdom have now been operating long enough for the strengths and weaknesses of the strategy to be clear. According to Gerry Stimson and his colleagues from the Centre for Research on Drugs and Health Behaviour who have kept a close eye on the UK programme, syringe exchanges have been particularly effective at reaching people not reached by more conventional drugs services. Around 60% of new clients at syringe exchanges say they have had no previous contact with any other drug project (52).

Exchanges answer a real need because the majority of clients are worried about scarcity of needles and syringes, and want to stop sharing because of fear of AIDS. They have also proved to be effective entry-points to other services, giving previously isolated drug users a place to get help and advice with a range of other concerns, from health care to housing, finance and the law.

By 1991, levels of needle-sharing in the United Kingdom had dropped to between a half and a third of the level found before the syringe exchange programme was introduced. Furthermore, needle-sharing levels are lower than those in countries, such as the USA, which do not have official syringe exchange schemes (53).

On the minus side, syringe exchanges in the United Kingdom are not working to capacity, and they are failing in particular to attract younger people, women, ethnic minorities, and those who have recently started injecting. Furthermore, they are having little success in en-

Comprehensive prevention: how many lives can it save?

We now know what works when it comes to preventing HIV infections: a basic package consisting of condom social marketing, STD treatment, AIDS information and education in schools and through the mass media, condom promotion for prostitutes and clients, safe blood supply, and needle-exchange programmes for drug users, all conducted within a supportive social environment. But what impact can prevention be expected to have?

AIDS prevention in a sense is more powerful than, say, cancer prevention. Preventing one HIV infection now will not simply prevent one death from AIDS, as preventing one incurable cancer would prevent one cancer death. Preventing an HIV infection now will help break the chain of epidemic transmission, averting the risk that the infected person will unknowingly pass the virus on to others who in turn might infect a still wider circle of people in the familiar "epidemic snowball".

This is why the impact of a basic HIV prevention package would be very large indeed. WHO has calculated that if comprehensive prevention were applied in all developing countries beginning in 1993, it could *halve the number of new adult infections* during the rest of this decade. This means saving the lives of almost 10 million people — over 4 million in Africa, over 4 million in Asia, and about 1 million in Latin America. But the ultimate saving in human lives would be even bigger because the main impact of reducing the epidemic snowball would be seen later, well into the twenty-first century.

couraging safer sexual behaviour, largely because the people who staff the exchanges, like their clients, find the subject of sex hard to bring up.

In the final analysis, syringe exchanges are only part of the answer to a highly complex problem, and in the United Kingdom there is a range of services and education initiatives. The emphasis of these programmes is to minimize the harm done by drug injecting — particularly the threat of HIV infection, but also such injection-related problems as abscesses, hepatitis B and endocarditis, all of which have decreased with the decline in the re-use of dirty needles.

As a first step to harm reduction there needs to be a shift away from emphasis on law enforcement, and towards making treatment and health and social services more available.

Thailand tackles its drug problem

After more than a decade of working with people dependent on drugs, the Health Bureau of Bangkok Metropolitan Administration (BMA) is acutely aware of how difficult it is for recovering drug users to return to a social environment in which they face all the pressures, frustrations and hopelessness that led to their drug dependence in the first place. More than three out of four people who complete detoxification courses at the BMA's narcotics clinics are back on drugs within months (54), a pattern that is fairly consistent worldwide.

Since 1985, both the BMA and a number of nongovernmental organizations have been running programmes for ex-drug users to help them find employment or to give them skills training that will allow them to work for themselves (55). Developing such initiatives became a matter of urgency when it became clear that drug-related AIDS was a serious problem.

Between 50 000 and 100 000 of Bangkok's 8 million people are dependent on drugs (56). The great majority inject heroin. The BMA set up 17 narcotics clinics after the extent of drug use became apparent in the 1970s — a period of rapid social and technological change that, Thai experts say, alienated many ordinary people (55). In 1988, serosurveys among clients of the clinics showed that HIV was spreading through the drug injecting population at a phenomenal rate. The first survey, conducted in January – March 1988, showed a seroprevalence of 15.6% — a figure that rose to 42.7% by the time of the second serosurvey, just six months later (57).

These alarming figures prompted the BMA to give special courses on AIDS to all clinic staff, and today AIDS programmes among injecting drug users consist of regular peer group counselling sessions for those who attend the clinics of their own accord — an average of 2000 – 3000 people a day — as well as outreach into the community to make contact with those not yet motivated to seek help.

"Rather than just giving instructions, we try to get groups to talk about their own concerns and to discuss the problem of AIDS themselves. That way we can learn about their habits and the best ways of helping them to change," said a social worker at one downtown clinic.

Equipped with a colourful flip chart giving the facts about HIV/AIDS, packets of bleach and a supply of condoms, she was leading a session with six young men and women. All watched intently as she showed how to mix bleach in the correct proportions and clean needles and syringes. Then came the discussion of safer sex. Smiles lit their faces as the social worker unrolled a condom and demonstrated how to put one on.

Among their peers, the clinic clients seem very ready to discuss their behaviour, the need for change, and how hard it is to alter one's lifestyle fundamentally. Here, too, the staff recognize the need to minimize the harm of drug use, in the face of AIDS, and not to insist on abstinence. The clinics now provide a number of treatment options ranging from a 45-day detoxification course based on replacing heroin with methadone in gradually diminishing doses, to promoting safer ways of administering heroin (e.g. by smoking), to meditation to reduce the need for a chemical high. "Addiction is a symptom of many causes, so there must be many responses," says Dr Suphak Vanichseni, deputy director of the BMA's health department. "We're doing research to determine the best forms of treatment. But addiction is not like malaria, which we can treat with one kind of pill."

Staff at the clinics take great pains to find the programme that is best suited to each client,

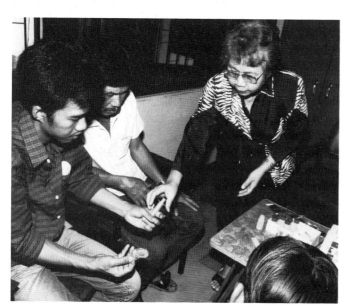

A social worker in a drug rehabilitation clinic in Bangkok gives clients information about AIDS. The group discusses the use of bleach to clean injecting equipment and the use of condoms for safer sex.

and to involve families in counselling too. Meanwhile, clients are encouraged to avoid needle-sharing or at least to inject more safely, after cleaning their equipment with bleach. "We believe there is less reliance today on the 'shooting galleries' where dealers inject drugs for their clients using the same equipment on many people", says the Director of the BMA's Health Department, Dr N. Choopanya.

The success of the clinic-based programme depends heavily on an agreement with the police that they will not arrest clients visiting the clinic — a fear that prevents many drug-takers from coming forward. This is not something that can be agreed once and for all, but a subject that needs constant negotiation with the police, says Dr Choopanya.

Community health workers, and a brigade of peer educators with personal knowledge of the drug scene, contact drug injectors who do not come voluntarily for treatment, providing them with information, bleach and condoms. Mrs Boouma Sua Wong, who runs a bakery in the working-class district of Suan Oy, has been a village health volunteer for over five years. Her face is familiar in the small, slatted wooden houses and narrow streets of the suburb where her job has been to encourage pregnant women to go for antenatal care, to weigh babies, advise on feeding, and remind their mothers to have them immunized. She administers first aid, too, from the small supply of plasters and pills provided by the health centre. But over recent years Mrs Sua Wong has been most preoccupied with spreading awareness of AIDS.

Besides her first aid kit she carries information leaflets, packets of condoms, and bleach, as she gathers people around her at any opportunity to talk, demonstrate, and hand out supplies. Does she know of many people who take drugs in her area? She nods her head vigorously. "I encourage them to attend the narcotics clinic," she says. "But if they're reluctant, I show them myself how to use bleach and send them away with some packets. I usually give them extra bleach and ask them to show their friends, because there are many drug users here who won't show their faces."

Mrs Sua Wong believes her work does have an impact in her small corner of Bangkok. "People are very worried about AIDS now and they listen to what I say, though they didn't believe it at first. But not many people come

A network of syringe exchanges

In Sydney, Australia, a syringe exchange was started in 1988 on the same premises as an official methadone clinic. From the beginning, demand for its services was so great that the authorities decided to seek changes in laws that were proving obstructive, and to expand the programme. At that time, anyone found in possession of drug-injecting equipment was liable to prosecution, which discouraged attendance at programmes for drug users. And only certain health officials had the authority to distribute needles and syringes within the mainstream public health system. Both these regulations have been changed and today a number of syringe exchanges, funded by health authorities, have established their own networks of satellite exchanges in New South Wales. They operate from a variety of outlets including clinics and mobile units.

Pharmacies have a complementary programme whereby they sell special low-cost packs containing a number of syringes as well as information on AIDS and safe injecting behaviour. To encourage safe disposal of equipment, specially designed bins, which cannot be reached into, have been placed in some public parks in a number of cities and towns.

Recognizing that injecting drug users are not a homogeneous and easily identified population group, the New South Wales AIDS Bureau of the department of health has worked hard to reach all kinds of people with information and encouragement to use the syringe exchanges. As word has spread to previously unreached networks of drug users, a number of exchanges have seen big increases in attendance.

An assessment of Sydney's programme in 1989 suggested that some 9–12 million needles and syringes a year would have to be distributed to meet the need for sterile equipment. By 1993 the programme was distributing around 3 million syringes, and some exchanges in the suburbs of Sydney as well as in the city centre were seeing attendances rise by 1000 clients per month from late 1992.

The increase in HIV infection rates among Australia's injecting drug users that was predicted early in the epidemic has never materialized: HIV prevalence in this population remains steady at below 5%. However, it is not possible to say how much the exchange programme has contributed to this picture, though it is undoubtedly meeting a need. While research into drug use among Australians had been occurring before the HIV epidemic started, there were no baseline data on injecting behaviour. Studies have now been commissioned to monitor HIV seroprevalence among drug injectors.

to ask for condoms, so I go out to visit people I think are at risk in their homes,'' she says.

Measuring the overall effectiveness of the BMA's AIDS prevention programme among injecting drug users is extremely difficult, but serosurveys indicate that the prevalence of HIV among clients of the narcotics clinics has stabilized at around 40%.

However, the programme has had less success with peer education than anticipated. By 1991, several hundred former drug users had been trained in health education workshops and given a small stipend for seeking out hidden drug users to provide them with AIDS information, condoms and bleach. They were supposed to report each month to the clinic staff, but many failed to turn up after a few months of work. ''The drop-out rate is about 50%,'' says Dr Suphak Vanichseni. One problem is that many get involved in taking drugs again when they come in contact with other users, a problem that drug outreach projects in many countries have faced.

Another programme found it hard to recruit former drug users for outreach because such people did not want others to know they had used drugs, and they did not want reminders of their old situation.

Personal experience — a valuable but volatile commodity

Despite the problems highlighted by Thailand's experiences, people who have themselves taken drugs play an active and valuable role in the fight against AIDS in many countries. They act as expert consultants to organizations designing programmes and information materials, and as peer educators and outreach workers where their personal experience makes them more readily accepted and respected than anyone from outside the drug-taking community. But the collective experience of such projects in many countries suggests that strong support, close supervision, and realistic expectations are essential to success.

''An important lesson we've learnt is that ex-users and current drug users are often willing to take on this responsibility because they see AIDS as a serious problem. But getting a project off the ground can be a difficult process,'' says Jo Kittelsen. ''People who are active users or who have just come off drugs are often very vulnerable people, and they're not used to being in control or to interacting with public or health officials on an equal footing. On the other hand, having a new source of income and a structure to life can sometimes help people to reduce their dependence on drugs.''

There are grounds for hope. Some studies have found high levels of AIDS awareness among drug users, an increased demand for sterile equipment, including an increased use of bleach, and a reduction in the sharing of needles and syringes. There is evidence, too, of changes in the social etiquette of drug taking in some countries so that needle-sharing is no longer seen as *normal* behaviour, but as an *exceptional* response to an emergency.

But despite all that has been learnt about successful strategies for prevention, the stigma attached to drug taking continues to frustrate efforts to control the drug-related spread of HIV. In many countries, politicians continue to emphasize criminal prosecution over social support, driving drug users underground and out of the reach of AIDS prevention programmes. Until they recognize that drug taking is a social problem, rather than simply a legal and policing one, and until tried and tested methods of prevention emphasizing harm reduction are used, vulnerable people — drug users and their partners, and *their* partners in turn — will continue to die.

CHAPTER 21

Caring for people with AIDS

"I had very good support from my family. They said, 'You are part of the family, you are the son in the family, why should you be treated as a different person?' They make me think I am one of them, that I am still important in the family. And they make me feel that it's okay to have what I have, there's nothing wrong in it. It's just another disease that not many people know about." — *Imrat, Malaysia* (59)

Everywhere, the epidemic of disease is advancing like a tidal wave that has been gathering force. Nothing that is done in the field of prevention can stop the wave from breaking, as the millions who are already infected with HIV go on to develop AIDS. In the communities where the virus started spreading earliest, and where AIDS has already become part of everyday life, the need for care — often over a period of years — is challenging families, friends and health care systems. This chapter will describe how a few of these communities are coping with the challenge.

Taking care to the people

In the Kagera Region of the United Republic of Tanzania, on the western shore of Lake Victoria, nearly half of all hospital beds are filled with AIDS patients. In poor, remote corners of the land, many more people are suffering and dying of AIDS at home, without any contact with the health services. In 1990,

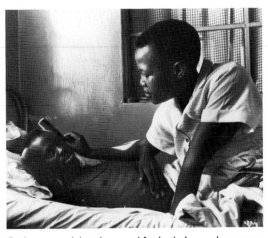

Patients too sick to be cared for in their own homes are admitted to Rubya Hospital. A family member is encouraged to accompany them, to help with the nursing and learn how to care for the patient once he or she returns home.

staff at Rubya Hospital, tucked away in a hilly rural area of the region and serving many villages round about, decided to try bringing clinical care to AIDS patients in their own homes as a way to ease pressure on the hospital and reach those who never came for treatment. Soon a small volunteer team consisting of two nurses and a clinician were bicycling or walking to see patients in the villages during their off-duty hours.

The team quickly realized that simple clinical care was not enough: patients and their families also needed some kind of counselling to help them come to terms with AIDS, their fears of death, and their anxieties about their children's future. So they appealed to WAMATA, a self-help organization for people with HIV/AIDS, to train them in counselling. Established in Dar es Salaam, WAMATA had recently started a branch in the Rubya area.

Under the guiding hand of WAMATA, Rubya Hospital's home-based care project won the backing of an international donor, becoming, in June 1991, the country's first pilot project for home-based care.

Today, the team consists of a paid administrator and assistant, besides the health professionals, who continue to volunteer their services free of charge. Every village in the project area has two or three village health workers (VHWs), all of them people with HIV infection or AIDS, who have been trained in basic health care, AIDS education and counselling skills. The project's eyes and ears at village level, the VHWs do what they can for people with AIDS and refer any problem they cannot handle to the professional volunteers. Patients too sick for home care are admitted to hospital, sometimes accompanied by a family member who is then taught how to care for the patient when discharged home.

Odelia Rwenyagira, a nurse-educator with the team, spends much of her time teaching home care to families and people in the community. She stresses good nutrition, the avoidance of opportunistic infections, and the pooling of resources to support families struggling with sickness and poverty. "We found that a lot of patients were dying not because of infections only, but because they were starving," says Mr Protase Karani, the project's administrator. "After prolonged illness when they couldn't work, they had nothing to subsist on. We talked to the community and got them to see that, rather than all contributing to the burial fund as is the tradition, they should contribute to looking after people with AIDS while they are still alive."

Besides the VHWs, other people with AIDS are also involved in the project as counsellors. "They are accepted easily by fellow patients because they have the same problems, and that's a big advantage in counselling," says Karani. "But working for the project helps the people with AIDS too: they get a small regular income; they get supplies from the project's small farm to keep up their strength; and because they're always in contact with us, they get early treatment whenever they have a health problem."

One problem the project has identified

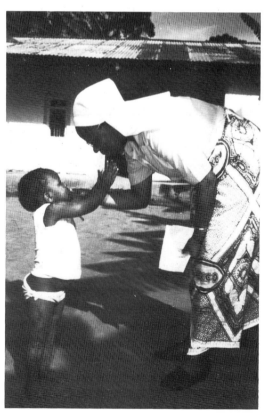

A child greets a member of the Rubya home-based care team in the traditional way — placing both hands against the visitor's cheeks.

is denial, even in the presence of debilitating symptoms. Walking along a path towards a house from which rose a plume of pungent wood-smoke, nurse Odelia told of the young woman she was about to visit, who was typical of the patients on her books. The woman had nursed her older sister — an AIDS patient — in Dar es Salaam until she died, only to return home sick herself. However, she would not acknowledge that she, too, had AIDS. "As long as they continue to deny their condition they're very hard to help," said Odelia. "Acceptance is one of the most important elements in treatment. But we don't push them. Perhaps after two or three visits this young woman will trust us and open up."

Rubya's home-based care programme has answered a real need. "If WAMATA hadn't been there I would already be dead. I had lost the will to live," says Dominic France, a father of seven who survived tuberculosis and now works as a peer counsellor when he is not troubled by swollen legs. His testimony is echoed by many in the hills near Rubya, where people who were wasting away from lack of care, hunger and despair have been thrown a lifeline.

However, there are many more who live beyond the scope of the programme. Thirty-six villages were originally involved in the home-based care scheme, but when it was chosen as a pilot project to be funded by foreign aid, the donor agency would cover only a few of the villages. "Being left out of the pilot study was a terrible blow to those communities," says nurse Odelia. "People became badly demoralized and most have gradually given up the struggle to organize self-help."

The mushrooming workload on the now tiny programme imposes a heavy strain, says Protase Karani. Having started with only 23 patients, the project had 227 people on its books within 18 months. The demand for counselling is such that patients seek out the project team at the hospital if they need to talk, rather than wait for their visit. The strains are exacerbated by the deepening poverty of the community, as more people become ill and die, leaving fewer and fewer resources on which to draw.

"The village government is supposed to pay the VHWs. But the village doesn't have money, so the project is paying a small honorarium to prevent them from becoming demoralized," says Karani. "WAMATA also has a

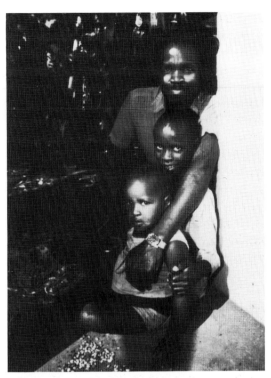

Dominic France, a man with AIDS and father of seven, had retreated from the world and lost the will to live until he joined a self-help organization. He became a peer counsellor, helping others with AIDS to overcome the kind of despair he knew well.

revolving loan scheme and VHWs are given priority in recognition of their work. We are also hoping to get them bicycles because they often have a long way to travel."

The model's reliance on low-paid or voluntary work, though unavoidable in most countries, could be one of its main drawbacks. A social worker in the regional capital, Bukoba, tried to sell the idea of home-based care to a gathering of "Ten Cell" leaders — officials of the lowest tier of the Tanzanian government who are responsible for ten households each. One man, who had been listening carefully, asked: "Who is going to run this thing? This is 1992, times are hard, who can afford to work for nothing?" He sat down to a round of applause from his fellow officials, who looked expectantly at the social worker for an answer.

But despite scepticism from some quarters, home-based care programmes — heavily reliant on volunteers from the communities served — operate successfully in a number of African countries including Kenya, Zambia, Zimbabwe and, most notably, Uganda, where The AIDS Service Organisation (TASO) was the pioneer in the field. The appeal of home-based care is that it uses the traditional care network

in rural Africa, the extended family, while providing professional support to help families shoulder the extra burden of AIDS (58). The burden falls mainly on women, who are the family's traditional care-givers.

Dr Roland Swai, head of the Tanzanian national AIDS programme, says the government is aware that hospitals could not cope alone with the burden of AIDS. "Treating chronically ill people gets cheaper the closer to the community you can deliver care," he said. "And with AIDS, care in the community is feasible. Families can do a lot if they are supported."

Women organize to help themselves

In the developed world, the majority of people with AIDS still look to mainstream health services for treatment of their opportunistic infections and other conditions. But the need for psychological and emotional support is increasingly being met by organizations outside the system — by support groups, hospices, and AIDS agencies set up at grass-roots level.

London's "Positively Women" is one such organization, begun in 1987 by a woman who found herself completely isolated after learning that she was HIV-positive. The only AIDS organizations in existence at that time had been set up by gay men; their perspective on the epidemic and the services they provided were naturally based on the experiences and needs of gay men. Women who came for help were frustrated by the lack of understanding of their circumstances. Some, for example, were mothers, anxious that their children would be taken away from them or subjected to discrimination at school.

There was also a great deal of denial in the developed countries that HIV was even a threat to women. Health personnel tended to be unsympathetic towards women who wanted to be tested for HIV, and sometimes incredibly insensitive when giving them their test results.

"I was told that I was a hysterical woman wasting National Health Service resources. After all 'women don't get AIDS, do they?'," recalls Kate Thomson, a founder member of Positively Women. A former drug user, she had gone for an HIV test hoping that her long history of drug-taking had left no lasting mark. "When the result came back positive, the doctor just said: 'You'd better not get pregnant because we've found antibodies to HIV in your blood'." Searching the shelves of bookshops for help and enlightenment, Thomson could find no women's faces in the literature on AIDS, so she answered an advertisement in the personal column of a feminist magazine for contact with seropositive women.

Most of Positively Women's early members had been infected through drug injecting, and the organization found it hard to get taken seriously or to attract funds because of prejudice about women drug users and concerns about their lack of work experience. But as the group became more effective, it received core funding from the British Government. In 1990 it was able to move from cramped spare rooms to its own spacious premises.

The old house in a quiet corner of London has been renovated using glass, wood, bright paint, and lots of green plants to create an environment that is restful and uplifting to enter. "We felt it was important for people burdened with their own problems to have somewhere nice to come to, rather than some grimy basement," says Thomson. "Also, one thing that comes up again and again is the importance of having a safe space, a place where a person doesn't have to hide her true identity or feelings, a place where women no longer have to live a lie." So, from the outside, the house is just one of the row with nothing to indicate its purpose.

Positively Women's clients come from all social backgrounds and circumstances: they have included university students, women in advertising, housewives, journalists, nurses, teachers and sex workers. Their common struggle with HIV and prejudice tends to bring social barriers down, but because of the diverse needs of people there are a number of different support groups to choose from. For example, there is a special group for African women who wish to discuss experiences specific to their communities. One-to-one peer support is available for women who are not ready to face a group, or for times of particular crisis.

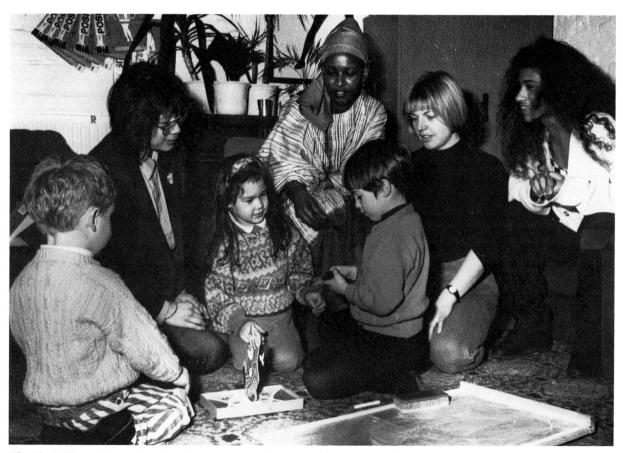

"Positively Women" organizes closed support groups for seropositive women only. But the organization also runs "open days" like this one, where staff, clients, friends and family meet to combat their isolation.

The project runs a telephone help-line and attempts to reach out to socially isolated women, for example minority or immigrant women, or those in prison. Clients are offered information and advice on welfare and benefits, and housing problems. And the organization offers professional massage to satisfy the deep need of HIV-positive people for physical contact. Advocacy for women at national and international level is another aspect of the group's work; members are often called on to speak in public or to provide technical assistance to other agencies.

An organization like this must have a clear idea of what it wants to achieve and why, says Kate Thomson. "You must decide how much you can handle because staff who take too much on their shoulders soon burn out. It's vital that there are mechanisms for staff support in place, because the work is emotionally very draining — helping people through sickness and death and seeing the anguish of their families."

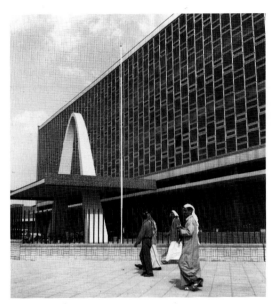

Ethical and religious principles in countries around the eastern Mediterranean call for people with AIDS to be treated compassionately and without discrimination, regardless of how they came to be infected.

What will become of my children?

In London, as elsewhere, women with HIV infection are wracked with anxiety about who will care for their children when they get sick or die. The problem is most acute for single women.

"Positive Options" was established in August 1991 by Barnardos, one of the UK's oldest and biggest children's charities. Research had shown that some family issues were being neglected by existing AIDS organizations. "Generally speaking, we found a lack of awareness about child-care issues among specialist HIV/AIDS workers, while child-care workers were often unaware of the issues surrounding AIDS," says Joan Fratter. Even when volunteers looked after children for sick parents, it tended to be an ad hoc arrangement, with few if any safeguards for the children's welfare.

Positive Options operates a scheme which sends child-care specialists on two-year secondments to work in existing AIDS organizations in the interests of children in AIDS-affected families. One such specialist is working with Positively Women; another is with Turning Point, a drugs and AIDS project; and a third

works with families affected by haemophilia and AIDS.

A second activity is the Planning Scheme, which operates out of the organization's own premises. A specially trained child-care officer helps parents with HIV infection to plan for the long-term future of their children, including who will care for them when the parent is sick or hospitalized, or simply in need of a break.

The ideal is for children to be cared for by a relative when the parents die, says Joan Fratter. But the stigma of AIDS and the overwhelming fear of rejection make it difficult for parents to explore these issues with anyone. Many have kept their status secret even from their families, and some are inhibited from talking to them because of the financial implications of taking on extra dependants. Dealing with these crippling inhibitions is often the first task of Positive Options.

Other options include fostering and adoption, and here all kinds of issues need discussing, says Fratter. "For example, one of our clients was a single mother with a very young child. She believed she had another two years of life ahead and she wanted to meet and get to know the family who would adopt her child. This is unusual but not unique. It means that a child can be helped through its bereavement by someone who cares and who has shared memories of the parent. Some continuity in life is preserved."

However, it is not just a matter of who will pick up the burden of care. There is also the question of how to prepare children for bereavement, and child-care officers encourage parents to make some personal record of their lives, and of their times with their children, to leave behind. Some parents have made video and audio recordings for their children; others have compiled photo albums or books of memories, and some have gathered objects of sentimental value into a box.

"Children often want to know things about themselves like what time they were born, the first words they spoke and when they took their first step. And they want to know about the history of their families," said Fratter. "We try to make parents aware of these needs of their children. But it can be a painful process and we let parents work through these things at their own pace."

Because of the expanding need for such a service and the pressure of work on the small staff, Positive Options sees its role as complementing the other kinds of long-term support offered to people with AIDS by counsellors, social workers and doctors.

Undoubtedly the availability of funds is an important consideration when it comes to the care and support of people with HIV infection and AIDS. But as these few examples show, it is not the only factor. Some of the most humane and caring systems have been established in the world's poorest countries, while some of the worst physical and psychological suffering has been allowed to occur in countries with money to spare. For effective programmes to be put in place, what appears most necessary is the determination to fight the stigma of AIDS that, in many places, still hides ordinary human faces and terrible human suffering.

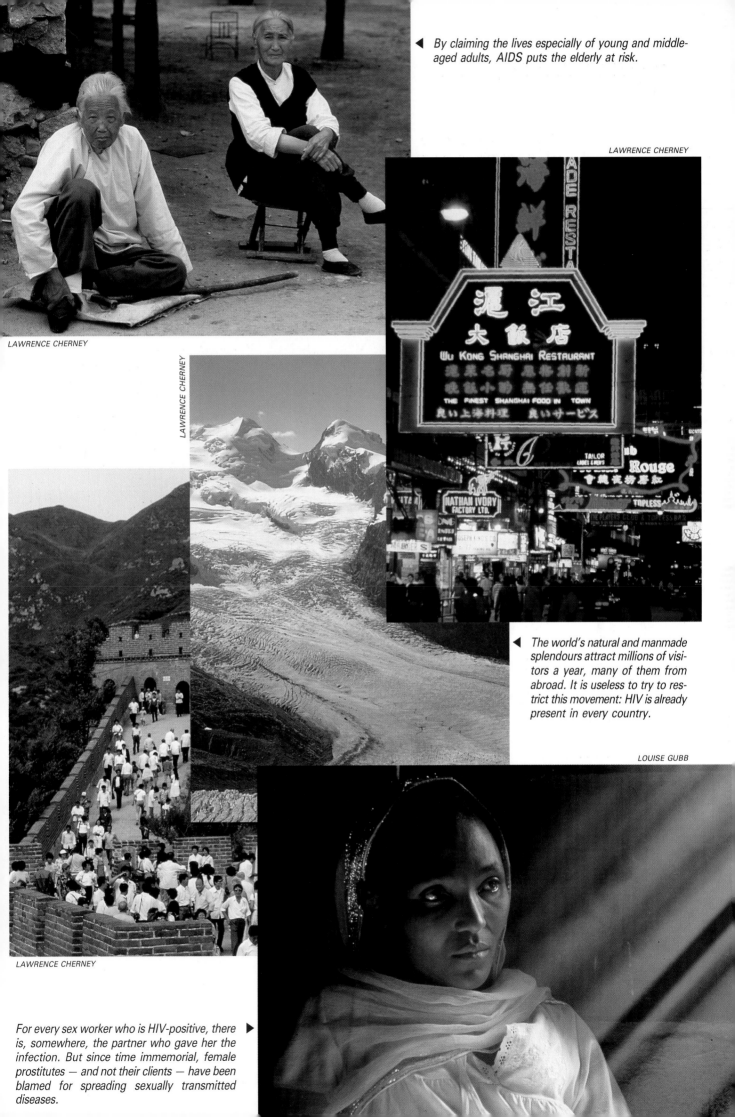

◄ By claiming the lives especially of young and middle-aged adults, AIDS puts the elderly at risk.

◄ The world's natural and manmade splendours attract millions of visitors a year, many of them from abroad. It is useless to try to restrict this movement: HIV is already present in every country.

For every sex worker who is HIV-positive, there ▶ is, somewhere, the partner who gave her the infection. But since time immemorial, female prostitutes — and not their clients — have been blamed for spreading sexually transmitted diseases.

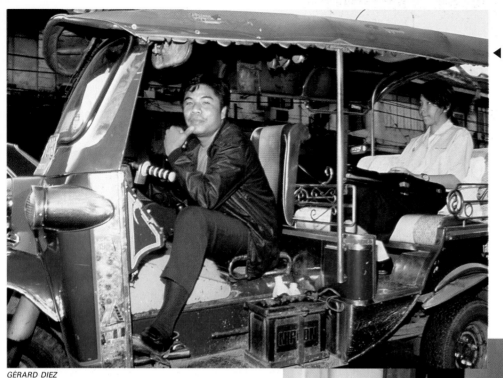

The popular tuk-tuks carry huge numbers of people around Thailand's towns and cities every day. Their drivers are ideally placed to pass on information about AIDS to the general public. In the northern city of Chiang Mai several tuk-tuk drivers have joined a network of volunteer educators.

GÉRARD DIEZ

A Tanzanian bar owner sees to it that her customers have easy access to protection from HIV. ▶

LOUISE GUBB

A wedding in a Tanzanian village in Kagera Region. Community leaders here, as in some neighbouring regions, have tried to curtail opportunities for sexual encounters by rescheduling weddings and other festive events to daylight hours.

FEDERAL OFFICE OF PUBLIC HEALTH, SWITZERLAND

Rester fidèle protège du s
les lettres d'amour déchir
quetées e
STO

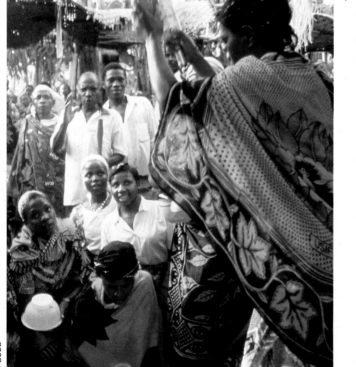

LOUISE GUBB

Dr Surasing, of the Provincial Medical Officer's office, has created and trained a network of volunteer educators at community level in Chiang Mai and surrounding towns. The volunteers,

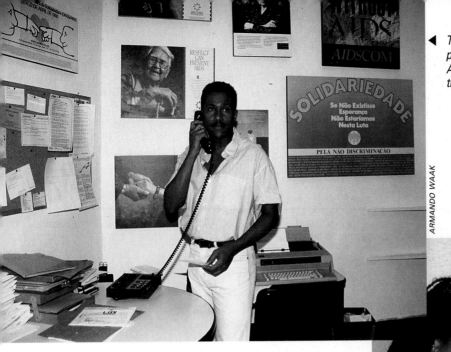

◄ Telephone hotlines, such as this one in Brazil, are popular ways of communicating information about AIDS. They give people a chance to air their anxieties and get their questions answered anonymously.

ARMANDO WAAK

Learning a skill gives women in Ethiopia some chance to get out of sex work if they want to, although it is hard to make a living from crafts.
▼

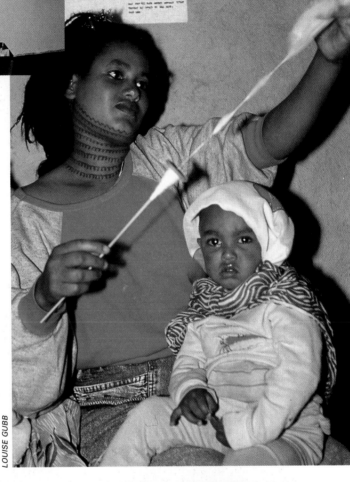

LOUISE GUBB

Protecting adolescents and adults from HIV is a matter of life or death. The surest way is to inform people about all the methods of preventing transmission so that they can choose the one best suited to their own circumstances. Here, a French poster playfully encourages condom use, while a Swiss poster reminds the viewer that fidelity helps prevent jealousy and torn love letters, not just AIDS.
▼ ▼

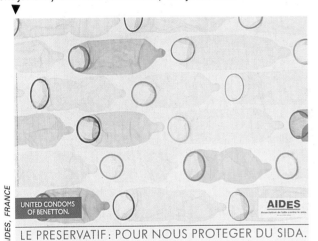

AIDES, FRANCE

UNITED CONDOMS OF BENETTON.

AIDES
Association de lutte contre le sida.

LE PRESERVATIF: POUR NOUS PROTEGER DU SIDA.

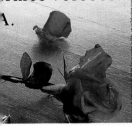

...us encore: fini
...photos déchi-
...rmes versées.
...1.

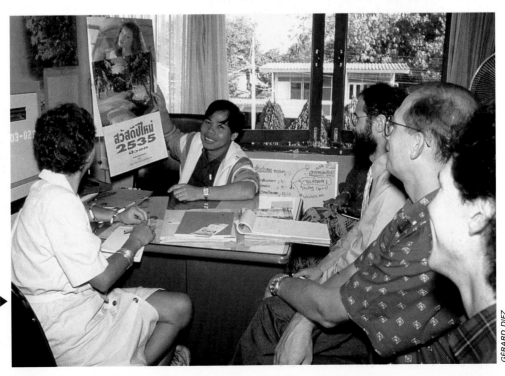

who provide AIDS informa- ►
tion to the general public,
include taxi drivers, hairdressers, and radio announcers.

GÉRARD DIEZ

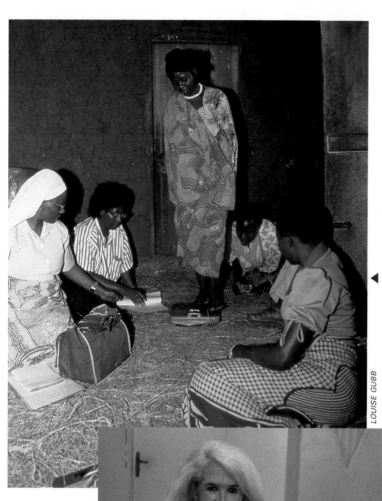

◀ Rubya's home-based care team visits a patient. Treating chronically ill patients in their own home is a particularly appropriate model of care for AIDS. Apart from cost considerations, patients are happier to be with their families, and families can do a lot if they are given professional support.

Brenda Lee, a travesti, runs a home for people with AIDS in São Paulo, Brazil.
▼

Community leaders in Bukoba, capital of Kagera Region, listen to a hospital social worker describe how home-based care for AIDS patients will work. The audience is sceptical about the scheme's reliance on unpaid volunteers. "Times are hard. Who can afford to work for nothing these days?" asks one man from the floor. ▶

Epilogue

Reactions to the AIDS epidemic show humankind at its worst and its best. In the same community where men will threaten their father's widow and children for standing between them and inheritance of land, a schoolteacher takes hungry orphans home for a meal and supplies condoms to bar girls and to boys approaching sexual maturity. In a slum where people with HIV commit suicide because of rejection by their neighbours, a housewife seeks out drug users to tell them about AIDS, distribute bleach and teach safe injecting practices. In a city where people receive scant hospital treatment because they cannot pay and are not insured, volunteers bring friendship and human warmth to HIV-positive babies confined to institutions.

As more and more people from all walks of life join a multisectoral response to AIDS, the twin priorities remain prevention of HIV infection and care of those infected. Preventive measures such as health education, condom promotion and protection of the blood supply have an effect all the way down the line.

But no matter how successful prevention efforts prove, care will become increasingly important because the world is only at the beginning of the epidemic of illness. The number of cases will spiral upwards for years to come as the millions already infected with HIV progress to AIDS. By the year 2000, the total will be more than four times what it is today.

While the achievements of the global response to date should not be underestimated, neither should the challenge ahead. AIDS is a catastrophe in slow motion, and it is essential that the world community pace itself for the long haul. The task ahead calls for clear vision, renewed will and greatly increased resources. But it also calls for greater determination than hitherto to use those resources in the interest of everyone: AIDS must not be allowed to join the list of problems, like poverty and hunger, that the world has learnt to live with because the powerful have lost interest, and the powerless have no choice.

References and notes

1. Cited in: Kolata G. AIDS researchers settle in for long haul. *International Herald Tribune,* 6 June 1991.

2. Mann J. *AIDS: a global report.* Address to the Conference on Integrated Strategy for Control of AIDS and Other Human Retroviral Infections and Hepatitis B, Tokyo, October 1987.

3. Personal testimony in: *America living with AIDS.* Report of the National Commission on AIDS, Washington, DC, 1991.

4. Armstrong S. Interview with Dr N. Clumek, *Economist development report,* August 1985.

5. European Study Group on Heterosexual Transmission of HIV. Comparison of female to male and male to female transmission of HIV in 563 stable couples. *British medical journal,* 1992, 304: 809-813.

6. Friedland G et al. Additional evidence for lack of transmission of HIV infection by close interpersonal (casual) contact. *AIDS,* 1990, 4:636-644.

7. Pietro Battiston is a person with AIDS who founded a hospice for AIDS patients in Johannesburg, South Africa.

8. Nakajima H. Address to the Sixth International Conference on AIDS in Africa, Dakar, Senegal, 1991.

9. Ungphakorn J. *The impact of AIDS on women in Thailand,* August 1990 (unpublished paper).

10. Stall R, Paul J. *Changes in sexual risk for infection with the HIV among gay and bisexual men in San Francisco.* San Francisco, Center for AIDS Prevention Studies, University of California, 1991.

11. Odelia Rwenyagira was a nurse-educator with Rubya Hospital's home-based care team, Kagera Region, United Republic of Tanzania, at the time she was interviewed.

12. Preble E. *AIDS orphans in Africa.* Paper presented to the meeting of Norwegian nongovernmental organizations on AIDS, Oslo, 4 December 1990.

13. Viravaidya M. *AIDS in the 1990s: meeting the challenge.* Address to the World Bank/IMF meeting, Bangkok, 12 October 1991.

14. Hanson K. *The economic impact of AIDS: an assessment of available evidence.* London, Health Policy Unit, London School of Hygiene and Tropical Medicine, 1992.

15. Viravaidya M, Obremskey S, Myers C. *The economic impact of AIDS on Thailand.* Bangkok, Population and Community Development Association, 1991.

16. Jonsen AR, Stryker, J, ed. *The social impact of AIDS in the United States.* Washington, DC, National Academy Press, 1993, p.5.

17. Merson MH. Address at closing ceremony of the VIII International Conference on AIDS/III STD World Congress, Amsterdam, 24 July 1992.

18. De Bruyn M. Women and AIDS in developing countries. *Social science and medicine,* 1992, 34 (3): 249-262.

19. Testimony from BBC World Service Programme : *The female god and other forbidden fruit.* Produced by J. Anderson, December 1991.

20. Frankham J, Stronach I. *Making a drama out of a crisis.* Centre for Applied Research in Education, University of East Anglia, April 1990. (Cited in: *PWA's confront teen denial* - Special Report of WorldAIDS, March 1991.)

21. Personal testimony to a meeting of the National Medical and Dental Association of South Africa, Johannesburg, May 1989.

22. Human Rights Internet. *Double jeopardy — threat to life and human rights.* March 1990.

23. *The global AIDS strategy.* Geneva, World Health Organization, 1992 (WHO AIDS Series 11).

24. *WorldAIDS Briefing,* No. 20, March 1992.

25. Barnett T, Blaikie P. *AIDS in Africa: its present and future impact.* London, Belhaven Press, 1992.

26. *AIDS analysis Africa,* September/October 1991.

27. *America living with AIDS.* Report by the National Commission on AIDS, Washington, DC, 1991.

28. See, for example, Serrill MS. Defiling the children. *Time International,* No. 25, 21 June 1993 : 40-43.

29. Duong Quynh Hoa. Affaiblissement des idéaux, changement des valeurs : commercialisation du sexe dans le contexte mouvant de l'ouverture, au Vietnam. [Weakening ideals, changing values: the sex trade in the changing context of "openness" in Vietnam.] In: *Proceedings of the Brussels Conference on the Sex Trade and Human Rights,* 6 March 1993. UNESCO, International Federation of Human Rights, International Council of Women, French-speaking Community of Belgium (unpublished document). Dr Duong Quynh Hoa is Director, Viet Nam Centre for Paediatrics, Development and Health, Ho Chi Minh City.

30. Esu Williams E. Keynote address to the VIII International Conference on AIDS/III STD World Congress, Amsterdam, July 1992. Dr Esu Williams is President of the Society for Women and AIDS in Africa (SWAA).

31. Ross Frankson J. A challenge to the powerless. In: Reid E, ed. *Reflections,* New York, Kumarian Press (in press).

32. Berer M, Ray S. *Women and HIV/AIDS. An international resource book.* London, Pandora, 1993.

33. Bledsoe D. The politics of AIDS, condoms and heterosexual relations in Africa: recent evidence from the local print media. In: Penn Handwerker P, ed. *Births and power: social change and the politics of reproduction.* Boulder, San Francisco & London, Westview Press, 1990.

34. AIDS: where do we stand, Lesotho? *AIDS,* magazine issued by the National AIDS Prevention and Control Programme, 1993, p. 4.

35. Zwi AB, Cabral AJR. Identifying high risk situations for preventing AIDS. *British medical journal,* 1991, 303 (6816): 1527-1529.

36. Ramalingaswami V. *The implications of AIDS in developing countries.* Address to the Sixth International Conference on AIDS, Florence, Italy, 1991. Professor Ramalingaswami is Professor Emeritus, All India Institute of Medical Sciences.

37. Ankrah EM. The impact of AIDS on social, economic, health and welfare systems. Plenary lecture at the VII International Conference on AIDS, Florence, June 1991. In: Giraldo G et al., ed. *Science challenging AIDS,* Basel, Karger, 1992, p. 186. Professor Ankrah is a United States national by birth, Ghanaian by marriage, and a permanent resident of Uganda.

38. Neequaye A. Prostitution in Accra. In: Plant M, ed. *AIDS, drugs, and prostitution.* London, Routledge, 1990.

39. Sebastian A. Report to the AIDS Council of South Australia's Management Committee on the Sex Industry Peer Education Project, January 1990.

40. Global Programme on AIDS. *Effective approaches to AIDS prevention.* Geneva, World Health Organization, 1993 (unpublished document WHO/GPA/IDS/93.1; available on request from Global Programme on AIDS, World Health Organization, 1211 Geneva 27, Switzerland).

41. Dowsett GW, Davies MD. *Transgression and intervention: homosexually active men and beats — a review of an Australian HIV/AIDS outreach prevention strategy.* Sydney, National Centre for HIV Social Research, Macquarie University, 1992.

42. Sabatier R. Crossing the threshold of fear. *AIDS watch,* No. 3, 1988.

43. *PWA's confront teen denial,* WorldAIDS Special Report, March 1991.

44. Defert D. Interviewed in *L'événement du jeudi,* 6 – 12 April 1989, p. 84. Daniel Defert, a sociologist, is the founder of the French organization AIDES and a member of WHO's Advisory Council on AIDS.

45. Green CP. *Male involvement programs in family planning: lessons learned and implications for AIDS prevention.* Study commissioned by WHO Global Programme on AIDS, June 1990.

46. Gordon G, Charnock D. Programmes to reach men. *AIDS watch,* 1990, 11.

47. Townsend S. Social marketing. *Network,* 1991, 12 (1).

48. *AIDS education and condom promotion for truck drivers, their assistants and sex partners in Tanzania.* Report by the African Medical and Research Foundation (AMREF), United Republic of Tanzania.

49. Serrano Y. Crackdown on AIDS. In: Rieder I, Ruppelt P. *Matters of life and death — women speak about AIDS.* London, Virago Press, 1989.

50. Stimson GV. Risk reduction by drug users with regard to HIV infection. *International review of psychiatry,* 1991, 3: 401-415.

51. Gruer L. *HIV infection and drug injecting in Glasgow.* Glasgow HIV/AIDS Resource Centre, Ruchill Hospital (unpublished document).

52. Stimson GV et al. In defense of legal syringe distribution: evidence from England. In: *Civil remedies in drug enforcement report,* Washington, DC, National Association of Attorneys General, December/January 1992, p. 19.

53. Centre for Research on Drugs and Health Behaviour. *Annual report 1991.* London, 1991.

54. Vanichseni S et al. A controlled trial of methadone maintenance in a population of intravenous drug users in Bangkok: implications for prevention of HIV. *International journal of the addictions,* 1991, 26 (12): 1313-1320.

55. Drug Abuse Prevention and Treatment Division. *Annual report 1989.* Bangkok Metropolitan Administration, 1989.

56. Vanichseni S, Choopanya K et al. *First seroprevalence survey of intravenous drug users in Bangkok, Thailand.* 1992 (unpublished paper).

57. Bangkok Metropolitan Administration. *AIDS prevention and control activities* (unpublished document).

58. Williams G, Campbell I. *AIDS management: an integrated approach.* Oxford, ActionAID, AMREF and World In Need, 1990 (Strategies for Hope, No. 3).

59. Personal testimony in: Richardson A, Bolle D. *Wise before their time: people with AIDS and HIV talk about their lives.* London, Fount Paperbacks, 1992, p. 108. Imrat is not his real name.

Photo credits

Country data by WHO region

The following tables have been compiled from answers to a GPA questionnaire sent to countries in late 1992, from other information supplied by countries, and from authoritative publications. The sources for all the information are stated in foonotes.

The symbol "−" denotes that the question is inapplicable or that information is either unavailable or not supplied.

The African Region

Table 1
Country information

	Total population (thousands)[a]	Population 0-14 years (%)[a]	Population 15-49 years (%)[a]	Population > 50 years (%)[a]	Annual growth rate (%)[b]	Urban population (thousands)[b]	Infant mortality rate[b, c]	Life expectancy men[b]	Life expectancy women[b]	Gross national product per capita (US$)[d]	Male literacy rate in 1990[e]	Female literacy rate in 1990[e]
Algeria	27 070	42	47	10	2.7	14 657	60	65	68	2 060	70	46
Angola	10 276	47	43	10	3.7	3 145	123	45	48	—	56	29
Benin	5 075	47	43	9	3.1	2 044	87	45	48	360	32	16
Botswana	1 352	45	45	9	2.9	383	59	58	64	2 040	84	65
Burkina Faso	9 788	45	45	11	2.8	1 727	117	47	50	330	28	9
Burundi	5 995	46	45	9	2.9	345	105	46	50	210	61	40
Cameroon	12 547	44	45	11	2.8	5 392	62	55	58	960	67	43
Cape Verde	395	44	46	11	2.9	121	39	67	69	—	—	—
Central African Republic	3 258	45	44	12	2.6	1 597	104	45	49	390	52	25
Chad	6 010	43	45	11	2.7	2 092	121	46	49	190	42	18
Comoros	607	49	43	8	3.7	179	88	56	57	—	—	—
Congo	2 441	46	44	10	3.0	1 030	82	49	54	1 010	70	44
Côte d'Ivoire	13 397	49	42	9	3.7	5 657	90	50	53	750	67	40
Equatorial Guinea	379	43	45	12	2.5	113	116	47	50	—	—	—
Ethiopia	54 628	46	44	10	3.0	7 058	121	46	49	120	—	—
Gabon	1 279	34	49	17	3.3	617	93	52	55	3 330	74	49
Gambia	932	44	45	11	2.6	226	131	44	47	—	39	16
Ghana	16 446	45	45	9	3.0	5 811	80	54	58	390	70	51
Guinea-Bissau	1 028	41	46	13	2.1	218	139	42	45	—	50	24
Kenya	26 090	48	44	8	3.3	6 766	65	57	61	370	80	59
Lesotho	1 882	41	46	12	2.5	405	78	58	63	530	—	—
Madagascar	13 259	46	45	10	3.3	3 412	109	54	57	230	88	73
Malawi	10 694	49	42	9	3.2	1 356	141	44	45	200	—	—
Mauritius	1 109	28	57	15	1.0	450	21	67	74	2 250	—	—
Mozambique	15 322	45	45	11	2.9	4 796	145	45	49	80	45	21
Namibia	1 584	45	45	11	3.2	469	69	58	60	—	—	—
Niger	8 529	48	43	9	3.3	1 838	123	45	48	310	40	17
Nigeria	119 328	47	44	9	3.1	44 802	95	51	55	290	62	40
Rwanda	7 789	50	42	8	3.4	457	110	45	48	310	64	37
Senegal	7 948	45	45	10	2.7	3 279	79	49	51	710	52	25
Sierra Leone	4 494	45	45	11	2.6	1 552	142	42	45	240	31	11
Swaziland	814	43	47	10	2.7	237	72	57	60	—	—	—
Togo	3 885	46	44	10	3.2	1 160	84	53	57	410	56	31
Uganda	19 246	49	44	8	3.0	2 300	103	41	43	220	62	35
United Republic of Tanzania	28 783	48	44	9	3.3	6 573	101	49	52	110	—	—
Zaire	41 166	48	43	9	3.2	11 789	92	50	53	220	84	61
Zambia	8 885	48	44	8	2.8	3 778	84	43	45	420	81	65
Zimbabwe	10 898	45	47	9	2.9	3 332	59	54	57	640	74	60

[a] Estimate for 1993. Source: UN Population Division 1992.
[b] WHO estimate for 1993 based on data from UN Population Division 1992.
[c] Per 1000 live births.

[d] Data for 1990. Source: World Bank (STARS) (April 1992).
[e] Source: Statistical Yearbook (UNESCO, 1991).

Table 2
Reporting of HIV and AIDS

	HIV infection first reported[a]	No. of AIDS cases reported		Cumulative no. of AIDS cases reported by 1 July 1993[b]
		1991[b]	1992[b]	
Algeria	1985	32	40	138
Angola	1985	130	187	608
Benin	1985	113	218	465
Botswana	1985	—	189	439
Burkina Faso	1986	—	0	1 307
Burundi	1983	1 565	1 583	7 131
Cameroon	1985	510	1 347	2 174
Cape Verde	1986	13	13	65
Central African Republic	1984	840	416	3 730
Chad	—	94	363	899
Comoros	1988	1	0	3
Congo	1986	1 077	1 785	5 267
Côte d'Ivoire	1985	3 894	3 863	14 655
Equatorial Guinea	1988	2	12	31
Ethiopia	1984	924	3 230	4 861
Gabon	1986	98	177	392
Gambia	1986	56	56	240
Ghana	1986	903	2 699	10 285
Guinea-Bissau	1989	30	116	288
Kenya	1980[c]	9 202	6 762	31 185
Lesotho	1986	28	131	219
Madagascar	1987	0	0	4
Malawi	1985	—	4 655	26 955
Mauritius	1987	—	6	16
Mozambique	1986	178	322	737
Namibia	1986	—	0	311
Niger	1987	212	290	795
Nigeria	1986	57	225	552
Rwanda	1983	—	2 908	9 486
Senegal	1986	125	323	911
Seychelles	1987	0	1	1
Sierra Leone	1987	52	32	95
Swaziland	1986	92	156	248
Togo	1987	628	675	1 953
Uganda	1983	8 706	4 421	34 611
United Republic of Tanzania	1983	12 059	4 579	38 719
Zaire	1986	3 120	1 181	21 008
Zambia	1985	1 646	1 276	7 124
Zimbabwe	1985	4 557	3 472	14 023

[a] Compiled from answers by countries to the GPA questionnaire.

[b] Based on other information reported to WHO/GPA by countries.

[c] HIV statistics.

[d] Sex not identified in 157 cases.

Table 3

The National AIDS Committee (NAC) and the National AIDS Programme (NAP)[a]

| | National AIDS Committee | | | |
	Year established	Chairman's position	NGOs represented (since)	Full-time NAP manager (since)
Algeria	1989	Medical Professor	no	no
Angola	—	Vice Minister of Health	—	1991
Benin	1987	Minister of Health	yes	1989
Botswana	1988	Permanent Secretary, Ministry of Health	yes	1992
Burkina Faso	1986	Minister of Health	1989	1989
Burundi	1988	Minister of Health	yes	1989
Cameroon	1985	Inspector General of Health	1985	1988
Cape Verde	1987	Medical doctor	yes	1988
Central African Republic	1986	Minister of Public Health and Social Affairs	1992	1987
Chad	1988	Minister of Public Health and Social Welfare	yes	1991
Comoros	1988	—	no	1990
Congo	1987	Minister of Health and Social Affairs	1990	1987
Côte d'Ivoire	1987	Minister of Health and Social Welfare	1991	1989
Equatorial Guinea	1988	Minister of Health	yes	1988
Ethiopia	1986[b]	Director of Armed Forces General Hospital	1989	1987
Gabon	1987	Minister of Health and Population	1990	1990
Gambia	1987	Director of Health Services	1987	1987
Ghana	1990	Medical doctor, private practitioner	1990	1987
Guinea-Bissau	1987	President of the Republic	1992	1992
Kenya	1985	Head of Microbiology Department, University of Nairobi	yes	1988
Lesotho	1985	Director of Laboratory Services	1985	1988
Madagascar	1990	Minister of Health	—	1989
Malawi	—	—	yes	1989
Mauritius	1987	Chief Medical Officer	1987	1991
Mozambique	1988	Deputy National Director of Health	1990	—
Namibia	—	—	1991	1991
Niger	1987	Minister of Public Health	no	1990
Nigeria	1988	Minister of Health and Social Services	1988	1988
Rwanda	1987	Prime Minister	yes	1989
Senegal	1986	Public Health Director	1986	1987
Seychelles	1987	Principal Secretary	no	—
Sierra Leone	1986	Chief Medical Officer	1987	1986
Swaziland	1987	Minister of Health	1987	1990
Togo	1987	Minister of Health	1990	1992
Uganda	1987	Minister of Health	1987	1987
United Republic of Tanzania	1989	Principal Secretary, Prime Minister's Office	no	1988
Zaire	1985	Minister of Public Health	1990	1988
Zambia	1989[c]	Deputy Director of Medical Services	1990	1990
Zimbabwe	1990	—	1990	1988

[a] Compiled from answers by countries to the GPA questionnaire, updated where possible by other information available to GPA in mid-1993.

[b] A Technical Advisory Committee.

[c] A National AIDS Committee was established but it was disbanded in 1990 and not reconstituted since. There is a management committee.

Table 4

Government departments and ministries implementing AIDS-related activities[a]

	Health	Education & culture	Social welfare & family affairs	Information & media	Interior, home affairs	Women & youth	Armed forces	Finance & planning	Labour	Other
Algeria	x	x		x		x				
Angola	x	x		x			x			
Benin	x	x	x	x						
Botswana	x	x								local govt lands & housing
Burkina Faso	x		x	x			x			
Burundi	x	x		x		x	x		x	
Cameroon	x	x		x		x	x			
Cape Verde	x					x				
Central African Republic	x	x	x	x		x	x			scientific research, international cooperation, rural development
Chad	x	—	—	—	—	—	—	—	—	—
Comoros	x					x				
Congo	x	x								
Côte d'Ivoire	x	x		x	x	x		x		
Equatorial Guinea	x	x				x				
Ethiopia	x	x	x	x	x	x	x	x		foreign affairs, tourism, agriculture
Gabon	x	x	x	x						
Gambia	x	—	—	—	—	—	—	—	—	
Ghana	x	x	x	x						
Guinea-Bissau	x	—	—	—	—	—	—	—	—	
Kenya	x	x								
Lesotho	x	x								
Madagascar	x	x		x	x		x			
Malawi	x	x	x	x		x				
Mauritius	x					x				family planning
Mozambique	x	—	—	—	—	—	—	—	—	
Namibia	x	x		x	x	x	x		x	agriculture, local govt & housing
Niger	x	x		x		x	x			
Nigeria	x	x		x		x	x			
Rwanda	x	x	x			x	x		x	
Senegal	x	x			x	x				tourism
Seychelles	x	x	x				x			
Sierra Leone	x	x	x							
Swaziland	x	x								
Togo	x	x								
Uganda	x	x	x	x	x	x	x	x		
United Republic of Tanzania	x	x		x						
Zaire	x	x	x	x		x	x			scientific research
Zambia	x	x					x	x		
Zimbabwe	x	x	x	x	x		x			agriculture

[a] Compiled from answers by countries to the GPA questionnaire.

Table 5
Supply of condoms

	Condoms distributed (thousands)[a]		Condom social marketing programme in 1992[b]
	1990	1991	
Algeria	—	—	no
Angola	—	—	no
Benin	400	550	yes
Botswana	—	2 000	yes
Burkina Faso	—	—	yes
Burundi	498	1 000	yes
Cameroon	2 160	2 160	yes
Cape Verde	—	—	no
Central African Republic	724	1 282	yes
Chad	74	444	no
Comoros	14	56	no
Congo	—	172	yes
Côte d'Ivoire	3 000	4 000	yes
Equatorial Guinea	288	288	no
Ethiopia	3 390	4 454	yes
Gabon	—	—	no
Gambia	576	834	no
Ghana	—	—	yes
Guinea-Bissau	—	114	no
Kenya	10 200	18 400	yes
Lesotho	367	502	yes
Madagascar	800	1 000	no
Malawi	5 000	5 000	yes
Mauritius	1 316	1 335	yes
Mozambique	2 370	2 592	no
Namibia	1 037	1 376	no
Niger		2 478[c]	no
Nigeria	1 000	750	yes
Rwanda	4 000	5 800	yes
Senegal	1 200	1 500	yes
Seychelles	100	309	no
Sierra Leone	1 008	1 500	yes
Swaziland	—	—	yes
Togo	—	251	yes
Uganda	—	1 800	yes
United Republic of Tanzania	20 000	30 852	yes
Zaire	4 140	18 715	yes
Zambia	—	—	yes
Zimbabwe	20 895	24 281	yes

[a] Compiled from answers by countries to the GPA questionnaire. The stated number of condoms distributed does not always include those sold by the private sector.

[b] Compiled from answers by countries to the GPA questionnaire and other information available to GPA.

[c] 1990 & 1991.

Table 6
AIDS information, education and communication (IEC)[a]

	AIDS & STD education included in school curricula (since)	Frequency of AIDS messages on:				Free air time given to AIDS messages			Promotion of condoms:	
		radio		television						
		more often than weekly	less often than weekly	more often than weekly	less often than weekly	yes	partly	no	through mass media	to vulnerable groups
Algeria	1992	x			x	x			yes	yes
Angola	no		x		x		x		yes	yes
Benin	no		x	x			x		yes	yes
Botswana	1992	x		—		x			yes	yes
Burkina Faso	1986	x			x		x		yes	yes
Burundi	1988	x			x		x		yes	yes
Cameroon	1991	x			x	x			yes	yes
Cape Verde	no	x			x		x		yes	yes
Central African Republic	1990	x			x		x		no	yes
Chad	no		x		x	x			no	yes
Comoros	no		x	—		x			yes	yes
Congo	1991	x		x				x	yes	no
Côte d'Ivoire	no		x		x	x			yes	yes
Equatorial Guinea	no	x		x			x		yes	yes
Ethiopia	no	x		x		x			yes	yes
Gabon	1990	x			x	x			yes	yes
Gambia	yes	x		—			x		yes	yes
Ghana	1991	x		x				x	yes	yes
Guinea-Bissau	no	x		—		x			yes	yes
Kenya	1992	x			x			x	no	yes
Lesotho	yes		x	—		x			yes	yes
Madagascar	1990		x		x	x			no	yes
Malawi	1991	x		—			x		yes	yes
Mauritius	no		x		x		x		yes	yes
Mozambique	no		x		x			x	yes	yes
Namibia	no	x		x			x		yes	yes
Niger	no	x		x			x		no	yes
Nigeria	no	—		—		—			—	—
Rwanda	no	x		—			x		yes	yes
Senegal	1991		x		x		x		yes	yes
Seychelles	1988		x	x		x			yes	yes
Sierra Leone	1990	x		—			x		yes	yes
Swaziland	1991	x		x		x			yes	yes
Togo	1982		x		x		x		yes	yes
Uganda	1989	x		x		x			no	yes
United Republic of Tanzania	no		x	—			x		yes	yes
Zaire	1988		x		x	x			no	yes
Zambia	1992	x		x			x		yes	yes
Zimbabwe	no	—		—			x		yes	yes

[a] Compiled from answers by countries to the GPA questionnaire.

Table 7
HIV antibody testing[a]

	Laboratory testing facilities at		
	central level	provincial level	district level
Algeria	x	x	
Angola	x	x	
Benin	x	x	
Botswana	x	x	x
Burkina Faso	x	x	x
Burundi	x	x	x
Cameroon	x	x	x
Cape Verde	x	x	
Central African Republic	x	x	
Chad	x	x	
Comoros	x	x	
Congo	x	x[b]	
Côte d'Ivoire	x	x	
Equatorial Guinea	x	x	
Ethiopia	x	x	x
Gabon	x	x	
Gambia	x	x	x
Ghana	x	x	x
Guinea-Bissau	x	x	
Kenya	x	x	x
Lesotho	x		
Madagascar	x	x	
Malawi	x	x	x
Mauritius	x		
Mozambique	x	x	
Namibia	x	x	x
Niger	x	x	
Nigeria	—	—	—
Rwanda	x	x	
Senegal	x	x	x
Seychelles	x		
Sierra Leone	x	x	x
Swaziland	x		
Togo	x	x	x
Uganda	x	x	x
United Republic of Tanzania	x	x	x
Zaire	x	x	x
Zambia	x	x	x
Zimbabwe	x	x	

[a] Compiled from answers by countries to the GPA questionnaire.
[b] In three regions.

The Region of the Americas

Table 1
Country information

	Total population (thousands) [a]	Population 0-14 years (%) [a]	Population 15-49 years (%) [a]	Population > 50 years (%) [a]	Annual growth rate (%) [b]	Urban population (thousands) [b]	Infant mortality rate [b, c]	Life expectancy men [b]	Life expectancy women [b]	Gross national product per capita (US$) [d]	Male literacy rate in 1990 [e]	Female literacy rate in 1990 [e]
Antigua and Barbuda	16 446	45	45	9	3.0	5 811	80	54	58	—	—	—
Argentina	33 487	29	49	22	1.2	29 092	29	68	75	2 370	96	95
Bahamas	268	28	58	13	1.6	176	23	69	76	—	82	69
Barbados	260	24	54	22	0.3	121	10	73	78	—	—	—
Bolivia	7 705	40	48	12	2.4	4 083	84	59	64	630	85	71
Brazil	156 578	33	53	14	1.6	120 847	56	64	69	2 680	83	80
Canada	27 755	21	54	26	1.4	21 581	7	74	81	20 470	—	—
Chile	13 813	31	53	16	1.5	11 786	17	69	76	1 940	94	93
Colombia	33 985	34	54	12	1.6	24 314	37	67	72	1 260	88	86
Costa Rica	3 270	36	52	13	2.4	1 587	14	74	79	1 900	93	93
Dominican Republic	7 621	37	52	11	2.0	4 782	56	66	70	830	85	82
Ecuador	11 310	38	51	11	2.3	6 646	57	65	69	980	88	84
El Salvador	5 517	42	47	12	2.2	2 526	45	64	69	1 110	76	70
Guatemala	10 029	45	45	10	2.9	4 075	48	63	68	900	63	47
Honduras	5 628	44	47	10	3.0	2 587	59	64	68	590	76	71
Jamaica	2 495	32	54	15	1.0	1 351	14	72	76	1 500	98	99
Panama	2 563	34	53	14	1.9	1 384	21	71	75	1 830	88	88
Paraguay	4 643	40	50	10	2.7	2 289	47	65	70	1 110	92	88
Trinidad and Tobago	1 279	34	51	14	1.1	841	18	69	74	—	—	—
United States of America	257 840	22	53	26	1.0	195 497	8	73	79	21 790	—	—
Uruguay	3 149	25	48	27	0.6	2 826	20	69	76	2 560	97	96
Venezuela	20 618	36	52	12	2.1	18 924	33	67	74	2 560	87	90

[a] Estimate for 1993. Source: UN Population Division 1992.
[b] WHO estimate for 1993 based on data from UN Population Division 1992.
[c] Per 1000 live births.
[d] Data for 1990. Source: World Bank (STARS) (April 1992).
[e] Source: Statistical Yearbook (UNESCO, 1991).

Table 2
Reporting of HIV and AIDS

	HIV infection first reported [a]	No. of AIDS cases reported		Cumulative no. of AIDS cases reported by 1 July 1993 [b]
		1991 [b]	1992 [b]	
Ahtigua and Barbuda	1985	6	0	6
Argentina	1982	478	605	2 456
Bahamas	1983	235	259	1 161
Barbados	1984	78	78	350
Belize	1985	11	12	53
Bolivia	1985	17	8	60
Brazil	1980	8 746	7 640	36 481
Canada	1982	1 006	931	7 770
Cayman Islands	1985	4	4	15
Chile	1984	177	162	723
Colombia	1983	782	434	2 957
Costa Rica	1983	84	117	470
Dominican Republic	1983	177	187	1 839
Ecuador	1984	51	57	253
El Salvador	1988	131	114	470
Grenada	1984	4	4	35
Guatemala	1984	95	94	434
Honduras	1985	495	709	2 510
Jamaica	1982	134	99	433
Montserrat	1989	0	0	1
Panama	1984	76	99	460
Paraguay	1986	10	18	56
Saint Lucia	1985	7	21	49
Trinidad and Tobago	1983	234	257	1 228
United States of America	1981 [c]	45 524	49 566	289 320
Uruguay	1983	86	90	359
Venezuela	1982	467	328	2 342

[a] Compiled from answers by countries to the GPA questionnaire.

[b] Based on other information reported to WHO/GPA by countries.

[c] 1981 is the year in which AIDS cases were first reported.

Table 3

The National AIDS Committee (NAC) and the National AIDS Programme (NAP)[a]

	National AIDS Committee			
	Year established	Chairman's position	NGOs represented (since)	Full-time NAP manager (since)
Antigua and Barbuda	1988	Chief Medical Officer	1988	1991
Argentina	1987[b]	—	1987	no
Bahamas	1989	National AIDS Programme Manager	1989	no
Barbados	1987	Professor in Medicine	1987	1992
Belize	1986	Programme Director	1986	—
Bolivia	1988	—	yes	1985
Brazil[c]	—	—	—	1990
Canada	1983	Director, British Columbia Centre for Excellence for HIV/AIDS	1990	no
Cayman Islands	1989	Medical Officer of Health	1989	no
Chile	1985	Undersecretary of Health	no	1991
Colombia	1991	Programme Coordinator	1991	no
Costa Rica	1985	Director General of Health	no	1987
Dominican Republic	1987	State Secretary of Public Health	no	1991
Ecuador	1989	Minister of Public Health	1990	1989
El Salvador	1990	Vice Minister of Public Health	no	1991
Grenada	1986	—	1986	1989
Guatemala	1984	Vice Minister of Health	1988	1992
Honduras	1987	Chief, Division of Epidemiology	no	1989
Jamaica	1988	Attorney-at-Law	1989	no
Montserrat	1989	Minister of Health	yes	no
Panama	1985	Minister of Health	yes	1989
Paraguay[c]	—	—	—	no
Saint Lucia	1986	Director, AIDS/STD Programme	1990	no
Trinidad and Tobago	1987	Chief Medical Officer	1987	1987
United States of America	1989[d]	Dean, School of Public Health, University of Michigan	1987	—[e]
Uruguay	1987	Vice Minister of Health	no	1991
Venezuela[f]	—	—	—	1990

[a] Compiled from answers by countries to the GPA questionnaire, updated where possible by other information available to GPA in mid-1993.

[b] Discontinued in 1990.

[c] There is no NAC.

[d] There was a Presidential Commission between 1987 and 1988.

[e] The National AIDS Program Office is headed by a Federal Coordinator.

[f] The NAC is not functional.

Table 4

Government departments and ministries implementing AIDS-related activities[a]

	Health	Education & culture	Social welfare & family affairs	Information & media	Interior, home affairs	Women & youth	Armed forces	Finance & planning	Labour	Other
Antigua and Barbuda	x									
Argentina	x	x							x	justice, municipality of Buenos Aires
Bahamas	x	x			x		x			customs department, police
Barbados	x	—	—	—	—	—	—	—	—	
Belize	x		x							National Drug Advisory Council
Bolivia	x	x			x					
Brazil	x	—	—	—	—	—	—	—	—	
Canada	x	—	—	—	—	—	—	—	—	
Cayman Islands	x	—	—	—	—	—	—	—	—	
Chile	x							x		
Colombia	x	x	x							
Costa Rica	x	x	x							justice
Dominican Republic	x		x				x			
Ecuador	x	x			x	x	x			
El Salvador	x	x	x				x			justice
Grenada	x	x						x		
Guatemala	x	x					x			
Honduras	x	x						x		
Jamaica	x	x	x			x		x	x	
Montserrat	x	—	—	—	—	—	—	—	—	
Panama	x	x								
Paraguay	x	x								
Saint Lucia	x	x	x		x	x			x	police
Trinidad and Tobago	x	x								Population Program Unit
United States of America	x	x	x		x[b]		x		x	justice, housing, veterans affairs
Uruguay	x	x								
Venezuela	x	x	x							IPAS/ME

[a] Compiled from answers by countries to the GPA questionnaire.

[b] States.

Table 5

Supply of condoms

	Condoms distributed (thousands)[a]		Condom social marketing programme in 1992[b]
	1990	1991	
Antigua and Barbuda	46	77	no
Argentina	—	—	no
Bahamas	—	30.5	no
Barbados	—	—	yes
Belize	108	173	no
Bolivia	300	200	yes
Brazil	—	7 000	yes
Canada	—	—	no
Cayman Islands	20	25	no
Chile	—	1 000	yes
Colombia	—	500	yes
Costa Rica	6 000	6 500	yes
Dominican Republic	50	50	yes
Ecuador	20	50	yes
El Salvador	—	—	yes
Grenada	230	250	yes
Guatemala	—	—	yes
Honduras	1 500	2 000	yes
Jamaica	—	8 500	yes
Montserrat	—	—	yes
Panama	—	—	yes
Paraguay	—	500	no
Saint Lucia	—	60[c]	no
Trinidad and Tobago	1 000	3 740	no
United States of America	—	—	no
Uruguay	450	800	no
Venezuela	2 000	2 500	no

[a] Compiled from answers by countries to the GPA questionnaire. The stated number of condoms distributed does not always include those sold by the private sector.

[b] Compiled from answers by countries to the GPA questionnaire and other information available to GPA.

[c] Distributed through maternal and child health and STD clinics. Figures are not available for January to June 1991.

Table 6
AIDS information, education and communication (IEC)[a]

| | AIDS & STD education included in school curricula (since) | Frequency of AIDS messages on: | | | | Free air time given to AIDS messages | | | Promotion of condoms: | |
| | | radio | | television | | | | | | |
		more often than weekly	less often than weekly	more often than weekly	less often than weekly	yes	partly	no	through mass media	to vulnerable groups
Antigua and Barbuda	no		x		x	x			no	yes
Argentina	1991	x		x				x	no	yes
Bahamas	1990	x			x		x		no	yes
Barbados	1988	x		x			x		yes	yes
Belize	no	x		x			x		yes	yes
Bolivia	no	x			x		x		yes	yes
Brazil	no		x		x	x			no	yes
Canada	1987	x		x			x		yes	yes
Cayman Islands	1988	x			x	x			no	yes
Chile	no	x		x				x	yes	yes
Colombia	1990		x		x			x	yes	yes
Costa Rica	no	x		x	—		x		yes	yes
Dominican Republic	no	—		—		—			—	—
Ecuador	no		x		x			x	yes	yes
El Salvador	1991			x				x	yes	yes
Grenada	1990	x		x			x		yes	yes
Guatemala	yes	x		—				x	no	yes
Honduras	1987	x		x			x		yes	yes
Jamaica	1992[b]	x		x				x	yes	yes
Montserrat	1992	x			x	x			no	yes
Panama	1991	x		—			x		yes	yes
Paraguay	no	x		x				x	yes	yes
Saint Lucia	1991	x		x			x		no[c]	yes
Trinidad and Tobago	1991	x		x		x			no	yes
United States of America	1987[d]	x		x		x			yes	yes
Uruguay	no	x		x				x	yes	yes
Venezuela	1991		x		x	x			no	yes

[a] Compiled from answers by countries to the GPA questionnaire.
[b] In 21 schools.
[c] Attempt stopped by the Church.
[d] In 80% of the states.

Table 7
HIV antibody testing[a]

	Laboratory testing facilities at		
	central level	provincial level	district level
Antigua and Barbuda	x		
Argentina	x	x	x
Bahamas	x	x	x
Barbados	x		
Belize	x		
Bolivia	x	x	
Brazil	x	x	x
Canada	x	x	x
Cayman Islands	x	x	
Chile	x	x	x
Colombia	x	x	
Costa Rica	x	x	x
Dominican Republic	x	x	x
Ecuador	x	x	x
El Salvador	x	x	x
Grenada	x		
Guatemala	x	x	x
Honduras	x	x	x
Jamaica	x	x	
Montserrat	x		
Panama	x	x	
Paraguay	x	x	x
Saint Lucia	x		
Trinidad and Tobago	x		
United States of America	x	x	x
Urugay	x	x	x
Venezuela	x	x	x

[a] Compiled from answers by countries to the GPA questionnaire.

The European Region

Table 1
Country information

	Total population (thousands)[a]	Population 0-14 years (%)[a]	Population 15-49 years (%)[a]	Population >50 years (%)[a]	Annual growth rate (%)[b]	Urban population (thousands)[b]	Infant mortality rate[b, c]	Life expectancy men[b]	Life expectancy women[b]	Gross national product per capita (US$)[d]	Male literacy rate in 1990[e]	Female literacy rate in 1990[e]
Albania	3 338	32	52	16	0.9	1 223	23	71	77	—	—	—
Austria	7 805	17	51	32	0.4	4 658	8	73	79	19 060	—	—
Azerbaijan	7 337	33	—	—	0.8	3 962	—	70[f]	70[f]	—	—	—
Belgium	10 010	18	50	32	0.1	9 656	8	73	79	15 540	—	—
Denmark	5 169	17	52	31	0.2	4 407	7	73	79	22 080	—	—
France	57 379	20	51	29	0.4	41 715	7	73	81	19 490	—	—
Germany	80 606	17	49	34	0.4	69 243	7	73	79	22 320	—	—
Hungary	10 493	19	50	31	−0.1	6 967	13	67	74	2 780	—	—
Israel	5 411	30	50	20	4.3	4 944	9	75	79	10 920	—	—
Italy	57 826	16	51	33	0.1	40 406	8	74	80	16 830	98	96
Latvia	2 669	22	48	31	−0.3	1 924	10	67	76	—	—	—
Lithuania	3 760	22	49	28	0.2	2 656	10	68	78	—	—	—
Luxembourg	380	17	51	31	0.7	325	8	72	79	—	—	—
Netherlands	15 270	18	54	28	0.7	13 564	7	74	81	17 320	—	—
Norway	4 310	19	51	30	0.5	3 285	7	74	81	23 120	—	—
Romania	23 377	23	50	27	0.3	12 899	22	67	73	1 640	—	—
Russian Federation	149 248	23	—	—	0.2	104 474	—	70[f]	70[f]	—	—	—
Spain	39 153	18	52	30	0.2	31 219	6	75	81	11 020	—	—
Sweden	8 692	18	48	33	0.5	7 337	5	75	81	23 660	—	—
Switzerland	6 862	17	51	32	0.7	4 319	7	75	81	32 680	—	—
Turkey	59 577	34	52	14	2.0	39 010	55	65	70	1 630	90	71
Ukraine	52 236	21	—	—	0.2	34 998	—	71[f]	71[f]	—	—	—
United Kingdom	57 826	19	49	31	0.2	51 635	7	74	79	16 100	—	—

[a] Estimate for 1993. Source: UN Population Division 1992.
[b] WHO estimate for 1993 based on data from UN Population Division 1992.
[c] Per 1000 live births.
[d] Data for 1990. Source: World Bank (STARS) (April 1992).
[e] Source: Statistical Yearbook (UNESCO, 1991).
[f] Figure does not differentiate by sex.

Table 2

Reporting of HIV and AIDS

	HIV infection first reported[a]	No. of AIDS cases reported		Cumulative no. of AIDS cases reported by 1 July 1993[b]
		1991[b]	1992[b]	
Albania	—	0	0	0
Austria	1985	176	170	943
Azerbaijan	1987	0	0	0
Belgium	1984	229	118	1 364
Croatia	1986	10	7	49
Czech Republic	1985	2	9	36
Denmark	1978	204	196	1 182
France	1982	4 248	4151	24 226
Germany	1980	1 450	1 286	9 697
Hungary	1985	31	32	120
Israel	1981	28	27	234
Italy	1982[c]	3 607	3 812	16 860
Latvia	1987	0	1	4
Lithuania	1988	0	0	3
Luxembourg	1984	12	12	62
Netherlands	1982	431	468	2 575
Norway	1982	60	50	319
Romania	1985	360	408	2 353
Russian Federation	1987	25	26	127
Slovakia	1985	0	0	6
Slovenia	1986	7	3	25
Spain	1981	3 469	3 469	18 347
Sweden	1985	137	119	817
Switzerland	1985	432	445	3 028
Turkey	1985	18	25	99
Ukraine	1987	3	4	14
United Kingdom	1982	1 810	1 268	7 341

[a] Compiled from answers by countries to the GPA questionnaire.

[b] Based on other information reported to WHO/GPA by countries.

[c] On stored sera, 1979.

Table 3

The National AIDS Committee (NAC) and the National AIDS Programme (NAP)[a]

	National AIDS Committee			
	Year established	Chairman's position	NGOs represented (since)	Full-time NAP manager (since)
Albania	1987	Minister of Health	1990	1991
Austria	1983	—	1985	—
Azerbaijan	—	—	—	—
Belgium	1988	Member of Medical Faculty	—	—
Croatia	1989	Minister of Health	no	—
Czech Republic	1990	Chief Public Health Officer	1990	no
Denmark	1986	—	1986	1986
France	—	—	—	yes
Germany	—	—	—	—
Hungary	1987	Chief, Division of Public Health and Epidemiology	1988	no
Israel	1986	Director General, Ministry of Health	no	no
Italy	1987	Minister of Health	yes	no
Latvia	—	—	—	—
Lithuania	—	—	no	1989
Luxembourg	1984	Directeur de Santé	1984	no
Netherlands	1985	—	1985	1985
Norway	1985[b]	Professor of Theology	1987	1985
Romania	1990	Minister of Health	1990	no
Russian Federation	—	—	—	—
Slovakia	1986	—	no	no
Slovenia	1985	Director General of the University Institute of Public and Social Welfare	1985	no
Spain	1987	General Secretary for Health	1988	1992
Sweden	1985[c]	—	—	1986
Switzerland	1988	Chief, Infectious Diseases	1988	yes
Turkey	1987[d]	Minister of Health	1992	no
Ukraine	1991	Member of Academy	—	no
United Kingdom	1985	Deputy Chief Medical Officer	no	1985

[a] Compiled from answers by countries to the GPA questionnaire, updated where possible by other information available to GPA in mid-1993.
[b] Reference Group for the Social and Health Departments.
[c] Abolished July 1992.
[d] Reorganized in 1993.

Table 4

Government departments and ministries implementing AIDS-related activities[a]

	Health	Education & culture	Social welfare & family affairs	Information & media	Interior, home affairs	Women & youth	Armed forces	Finance & planning	Labour	Other
Albania	x	x		x						
Austria	x									
Azerbaijan	x	–	–	–	–	–	–	–	–	
Belgium	x	–	–	–	–	–	–	–	–	
Croatia	x	x		x						
Czech Republic	x	x								
Denmark	x									countries, municipalities
France	x	x					x			agriculture, justice, local government, tourism
Germany	x	x								economic cooperation, research and technology
Hungary	x									
Israel	x	x	x				x			
Italy	x	–	–	–	–	–	–	–	–	
Latvia	x	–	–	–	–	–	–	–	–	
Lithuania	x			x						
Luxembourg	x	x	x							
Netherlands	x	x	x	x						justice, local government
Norway	x	x								
Romania	x	–	–	–	–	–	–	–	–	
Russian Federation	x	x	x	x						
Slovakia	x	x		x			x			
Slovenia	x	x		x						
Spain	x	x					x			justice
Sweden	x		x							
Switzerland	x	x								
Turkey	x	–	–	–	–	–	–	–	–	
Ukraine	x	–	–	–	–	–	–	–	–	
United Kingdom	x									local government

[a] Compiled from answers by countries to the GPA questionnaire.

Table 5
Supply of condoms

	Condoms distributed (thousands)[a]		Condom social marketing programme in 1992[b]
	1990	1991	
Albania	—	—	no
Austria	—	—	no
Azerbaijan	2 000	3 000	no
Belgium	10 000	10 000	yes
Croatia	—	—	no
Czech Republic	3 520	5 231	no
Denmark	—	14 000[c]	yes
France	70 000	92 000	yes
Germany	—	—	no
Hungary	15 000	18 000	yes
Israel	—	—	yes
Italy	—	—	no
Latvia	—	1 000	no
Lithuania	—	—	no
Luxembourg	—	—	no
Netherlands	390	350	no
Norway	9 951	8 937	yes
Romania	—	—	no
Russian Federation	—	—	yes
Slovakia	1 500	2 500	no
Slovenia	—	—	no
Spain	—	1 000	yes
Sweden	22 000	22 000	yes
Switzerland	12 700	13 800	yes
Turkey	13 452	12 264	yes
Ukraine	—	—	no
United Kingdom	145 000	148 000	no

[a] Compiled from answers by countries to the GPA questionnaire. The stated number of condoms distributed does not always include those sold by the private sector.

[b] Compiled from answers by countries to the GPA questionnaire and other information available to GPA. Some of the replies concerning "condom social marketing" pertain to condom promotion activities in general.

[c] 1990 and 1991.

Table 6
AIDS information, education and communication (IEC)[a]

	AIDS & STD education included in school curricula (since)	Frequency of AIDS messages on:				Free air time given to AIDS messages			Promotion of condoms:	
		radio		television						
		more often than weekly	less often than weekly	more often than weekly	less often than weekly	yes	partly	no	through mass media	to vulnerable groups
Albania	no		x		x	x			yes	yes
Austria	yes		x		x			x	yes	no
Azerbaijan	1990		x		x		x		no	yes
Belgium	yes		x		x		x		yes	yes
Croatia	1990		x		x		x		yes	no
Czech Republic	1991	x		x			x		yes	yes
Denmark	yes		x		x		x		yes	yes
France	1987		x		x		x		yes	yes
Germany	—	—		x		x			yes	yes
Hungary	no	x		x			x		yes	yes
Israel	yes		x		x	x			yes	yes
Italy	1993		x		x			x	yes	yes
Latvia	1990		x		x		x		yes	yes
Lithuania	no	x		x				x	yes	yes
Luxembourg	1988		x		x		x		no	yes
Netherlands	1991	x		x			x		yes	yes
Norway	1986		x		x	x			yes	yes
Romania	no		x		x		x		no	no
Russian Federation	1989		x		x		x		yes	yes
Slovakia	no		x		x	x			yes	yes
Slovenia	1989		x		x		x		yes	yes
Spain	1992	—		—			x		yes	yes
Sweden	1977		x		x			x	yes	yes
Switzerland	b	x		x			x		yes	yes
Turkey	no		x		x		x		no	no
Ukraine	—	x			x		x		yes	yes
United Kingdom	1992		x		x			x	yes	yes

[a] Compiled from answers by countries to the GPA questionnaire.
[b] Different in each canton.

Table 7
HIV antibody testing[a]

	Laboratory testing facilities at		
	central level	provincial level	district level
Albania	x		
Austria	x	x	x
Azerbaijan	x	x	x
Belgium	x	x	x
Croatia	x	x	x
Czech Republic	x	x	x
Denmark	x	x	x
France	x	x	x
Germany	x	x	x
Hungary	x	x	x
Israel	x	x	x
Italy	x	x	x
Latvia	x	x	x
Lithuania	x	x	x
Luxembourg	x	x	x
Netherlands	x	x	x
Norway	x	x	
Romania	x	x	x
Russian Federation	x	x	x
Slovakia	x	x	x
Slovenia	x	x	
Spain	x	x	x
Sweden	x	x	x
Switzerland	x	x	x
Turkey	x	x	
Ukraine	x	x	x
United Kingdom	x	x	x

[a] Compiled from answers by countries to the GPA questionnaire.

The Eastern Mediterranean Region

Table 1
Country information

	Total population (thousands)[a]	Population 0-14 years (%)[a]	Population 15-49 years (%)[a]	Population > 50 years (%)[a]	Annual growth rate (%)[b]	Urban population (thousands)[b]	Infant mortality rate[b, c]	Life expectancy men[b]	Life expectancy women[b]	Gross national product per capita (US$)[d]	Male literacy rate in 1990[e]	Female literacy rate in 1990[e]
Cyprus	723	26	51	23	0.9	396	9	75	79	—	—	—
Djibouti	481	46	45	10	3.0	394	111	48	51	—	—	—
Egypt	56 060	39	49	12	2.2	24 882	56	61	63	600	63	34
Iran (Islamic Republic of)	63 180	46	43	10	2.7	37 253	39	67	68	2 490	65	43
Iraq	19 918	44	47	9	3.2	14 629	57	65	68	—	70	49
Jordan	4 440	44	47	9	3.4	3 111	35	66	70	1 240	89	70
Kuwait	1 825	39	54	7	−5.1	1 739	14	73	78	—	77	67
Lebanon	2 901	34	51	14	2.0	2 496	34	67	71	—	88	73
Libyan Arab Jamahiriya	5 048	46	45	10	3.5	4 262	67	62	65	—	—	—
Morocco	26 954	39	49	11	2.4	12 778	67	62	65	950	61	38
Pakistan	128 057	44	47	9	2.7	42 986	97	59	59	380	47	21
Saudi Arabia	16 472	42	48	9	3.4	13 006	30	68	71	7 050	73	48
Sudan	13 762	48	44	8	3.6	7 081	39	65	69	1 000	78	51
Syrian Arab Republic	27 407	45	45	10	2.8	6 510	98	51	53	—	43	12
Tunisia	8 579	36	51	13	2.0	4 952	42	67	69	1 440	74	56
Yemen	12 977	50	42	8	3.5	4 104	105	52	53	—	53	26

[a] Estimate for 1993. Source: UN Population Division 1992.
[b] WHO estimate for 1993 based on data from UN Population Division 1992.
[c] Per 1000 live births.
[d] Data for 1990. Source: World Bank (STARS) (April 1992).
[e] Source: Statistical Yearbook (UNESCO, 1991).

Table 2

Reporting of HIV and AIDS

	HIV infection first reported[a]	No. of AIDS cases reported		Cumulative no. of AIDS cases reported by 1 July 1993[b]
		1991[b]	1992[b]	
Cyprus	1986	4	1	24
Djibouti	1986	107	144	355
Egypt	1986	12	23	64
Iran (Islamic Republic of)	1987	25	16	60
Iraq	1991[c]	25	6	31
Jordan	1986	6	7	27
Kuwait	1984	3	2	8
Lebanon	1984	7	6	44
Libyan Arab Jamahiriya	1986	2	3	10
Morocco	1986	28	30	145
Pakistan	1987	4	8	26
Saudi Arabia	1986	8	8	50
Sudan	1986	182	184	727
Syrian Arab Republic	1986	4	3	21
Tunisia	1985	28	25	126
Yemen	1989	2[d]	2	2

[a] Compiled from answers by countries to the GPA questionnaire.
[b] Based on other information reported to WHO/GPA by countries.
[c] 1989 — foreign visitors.
[d] According to the questionnaire, two people died from AIDS in 1991.

Table 3

The National AIDS Committee (NAC) and the National AIDS Programme (NAP)[a]

	National AIDS Committee			
	Year established	Chairman's position	NGOs represented (since)	Full-time NAP manager (since)
Cyprus	1986	Minister of Health	1986	no
Djibouti	1991	Technical Director, Ministry of Health	1991	no
Egypt	1986	Undersecretary of Preventive Affairs	1992	1990
Iran (Islamic Republic of)	1987	Undersecretary for Health Affairs	1991	1990
Iraq	1986	Director General of Preventive Medicine	1991	1987
Jordan	1986	Secretary General, Ministry of Health	1986	1991
Kuwait	1988	Undersecretary of Public Health	no	no
Lebanon	1988	General Director of Health	1992	1990
Libyan Arab Jamahiriya	1987	Undersecretary of Health	no	no
Morocco	1986	Director of Epidemiology and Sanitary Programme	1988	1988
Pakistan	—	Secretary of Health	1991	1990
Saudi Arabia	1986	Deputy Minister of Health for Executive Affairs	no	1986
Sudan	1987	Minister of Health[b]	1987	1990
Syrian Arab Republic	1988	Minister of Health	1988	no
Tunisia	1986	Minister of Public Health	no	no
Yemen	1989	Undersecretary of Health	no	1991

[a] Compiled from answers by countries to the GPA questionnaire, updated where possible by other information available to GPA in mid-1993.
[b] Patronage by the President of the Republic.

Table 4
Government departments and ministries implementing AIDS-related activities[a]

	Health	Education & culture	Social welfare & family affairs	Information & media	Interior, home affairs	Women & youth	Armed forces	Finance & planning	Labour	Other
Cyprus	x	x		x		x				
Djibouti	x			x		x				religous affairs
Egypt	x	x	x	x						
Iran (Islamic Republic of)	x									
Iraq	x	x		x		x	x			religous affairs
Jordan	x	x		x						
Kuwait	x									
Lebanon	x	x		x	x					
Libyan Arab Jamahiriya	x	x		x						justice
Morocco	x	—	—	—	—	—	—	—		
Pakistan	x			x	x					ministry of commerce
Saudi Arabia	x	x		x						
Sudan	x	x		x		x				
Syrian Arab Republic	x									
Tunisia	x	x		x	x					tourism
Yemen	x									

[a] Compiled from answers by countries to the GPA questionnaire.

Table 5
Supply of condoms

	Condoms distributed (thousands)[a]		Condom social marketing programme in 1992[b]
	1990	1991	
Cyprus	—	144	no
Djibouti	304	300	no
Egypt	—	20 000	yes
Iran (Islamic Republic of)	—	—	no
Iraq	0	0	no
Jordan	420	832	yes
Kuwait	0	0	no
Lebanon	500	500	no
Libyan Arab Jamahiriya	—	—	no
Morocco	1 722	3 312	yes
Pakistan	0	0	yes
Saudi Arabia	—	—	no
Sudan	20	20	no
Syrian Arab Republic	—	—	—
Tunisia	2 000	2 800	yes
Yemen	0	0	no

[a] Compiled from answers by countries to the GPA questionnaire. The stated number of condoms distributed does not always include those sold by the private sector.
[b] Compiled from answers by countries to the GPA questionnaire and other information available to GPA.

Table 6
AIDS information, education and communication (IEC)[a]

	AIDS & STD education included in school curricula (since)	Frequency of AIDS messages on:				Free air time given to AIDS messages			Promotion of condoms:	
		radio		television						
		more often than weekly	less often than weekly	more often than weekly	less often than weekly	yes	partly	no	through mass media	to vulnerable groups
Cyprus	1992	x		x		x			no	yes
Djibouti	no		x		x	x			no	yes
Egypt	no	x		x		x			yes	no
Iran (Islamic Republic of)	no		x		x			x	no	yes
Iraq	1991		x		x		x		no	yes
Jordan	no		x		x		x		no	no
Kuwait	1989	x		x		x			no	no
Lebanon	no		x		x	x			yes	no
Libyan Arab Jamahiriya	1989		x		x		x		no	yes
Morocco	1991		x		x		x		yes	no
Pakistan	no	—		—				x	yes	yes
Saudi Arabia	no		x		x			x	no	no
Sudan	1992	x			x		x		no	yes
Syrian Arab Republic	1990		x		x	x			no	yes
Tunisia	1989		x		x	x			yes[b]	yes
Yemen	no	—			x		x		no	yes

[a] Compiled from answers by countries to the GPA questionnaire.
[b] Essentially for family planning.

Table 7
HIV antibody testing[a]

	Laboratory testing facilities at		
	central level	provincial level	district level
Cyprus	x	x	x
Djibouti	x		
Egypt	x	x	
Iran (Islamic Republic of)	x	x	x
Iraq	x	x	
Jordan	x	x	
Kuwait	x		
Lebanon	x	x	
Libyan Arab Jamahiriya	x	x	
Morocco	x	x	
Pakistan	x	x	x
Saudi Arabia	x	x	x
Sudan	x	x	x
Syrian Arab Republic	x	x	
Tunisia	x	x	x
Yemen	x		

[a] Compiled from answers by countries to the GPA questionnaire.

The South-East Asia Region

Table 1
Country information

	Total population (thousands)[a]	Population 0-14 years (%)[a]	Population 15-49 years (%)[a]	Population >50 years (%)[a]	Annual growth rate (%)[b]	Urban population (thousands)[b]	Infant mortality rate[b,c]	Life expectancy men[b]	Life expectancy women[b]	Gross national product per capita (US$)[d]	Male literacy rate in 1990[e]	Female literacy rate in 1990[e]
Bangladesh	122 210	41	49	10	2.4	22 288	106	53	53	210	47	22
Bhutan	1 650	41	48	12	2.3	98	127	48	49	190	–	–
India	896 567	35	50	14	1.9	235 509	87	60	61	350	62	34
Indonesia	194 617	34	52	14	1.8	60 229	64	61	65	570	84	68
Maldives	234	44	45	11	3.0	74	53	65	62	–	–	–
Myanmar	44 613	38	50	13	2.1	11 421	80	56	60	–	89	72
Nepal	21 086	43	46	11	2.4	2 633	98	54	53	170	38	13
Sri Lanka	17 894	31	53	16	1.3	3 930	24	70	74	470	93	84
Thailand	56 868	30	56	13	1.2	13 661	26	67	72	1420	96	90

[a] Estimate for 1993. Source: UN Population Division 1992.
[b] WHO estimate for 1993 based on data from UN Population Division 1992.
[c] Per 1000 live births.
[d] Data for 1990. Source: World Bank (STARS) (April 1992).
[e] Source: Statistical Yearbook (UNESCO, 1991).

Table 2
Reporting of HIV and AIDS

	HIV infection first reported[a]	No. of AIDS cases reported 1991[b]	No. of AIDS cases reported 1992[b]	Cumulative no. of AIDS cases reported by 1 July 1993[b]
Bangladesh	1989	1	0	1
Bhutan	–	0	0	0
India	1986	45	140	312
Indonesia	1987	9	3	31
Maldives	1991	0	0	0
Myanmar	1988	6	6	47
Nepal	1988	4	3	18
Sri Lanka	1986	3	0	24
Thailand	1985	398	730	1569

[a] Compiled from answers by countries to the GPA questionnaire.
[b] Based on other information reported to WHO/GPA by countries.

Table 3
The National AIDS Committee (NAC) and the National AIDS Programme (NAP)[a]

| | National AIDS Committee | | | |
	Year established	Chairman's position	NGOs represented (since)	Full-time NAP manager (since)
Bangladesh	1985	Deputy Leader of Parliament	1992	no
Bhutan	1989	Deputy Minister of Social Services	1989	no
India	1992	Union Minister of Health and Family Welfare	1992	1992
Indonesia	1987	Director General of Health	1988	no
Maldives	1990	Medical Adviser, Ministry of Health and Welfare	—	no
Myanmar	1988	Minister of Health	1991	1991
Nepal	1990	Secretary of Health	1990	1992
Sri Lanka	1988[b]	Director General of Health	1988	no
Thailand	1988	Prime Minister	1988	1987

[a] Compiled from answers by countries to the GPA questionnaire, updated where possible by other information available to GPA in mid-1993.
[b] The Task Force (1986) was replaced by the NAC.

Table 4
Government departments and ministries implementing AIDS-related activities[a]

	Health	Education & culture	Social welfare & family affairs	Information & media	Interior, home affairs	Women & youth	Armed forces	Finance & planning	Labour	Other
Bangladesh	x									
Bhutan	x									
India	x	x								
Indonesia	x	x								
Maldives	x			x						
Myanmar	x	—	—	—	—	—	—	—	—	
Nepal	x									
Sri Lanka	x									
Thailand	x				x					Office of the Prime Minister

[a] Compiled from answers by countries to the GPA questionnaire.

Table 5
Supply of condoms

	Condoms distributed (thousands)[a]		Condom social marketing programme in 1992[b]
	1990	1991	
Bangladesh	—	—	yes
Bhutan	—	—	no
India	—	1 100 000	yes
Indonesia	50	25	yes
Maldives	0	0	no
Myanmar	—	29	no
Nepal	—	20	yes
Sri Lanka	0	80	yes
Thailand	14 443	31 950	yes

[a] Compiled from answers by countries to the GPA questionnaire. The stated number of condoms distributed does not always include those sold by the private sector.
[b] Compiled from answers by countries to the GPA questionnaire and other information available to GPA.

Table 6
AIDS information, education and communication (IEC)[a]

	AIDS & STD education included in school curricula (since)	Frequency of AIDS messages on:				Free air time given to AIDS messages			Promotion of condoms:	
		radio		television						
		more often than weekly	less often than weekly	more often than weekly	less often than weekly	yes	partly	no	through mass media	to vulnerable groups
Bangladesh	no		x		x		x		yes	no
Bhutan	no		x	—		x			no	yes
India	no	—			x		x		yes	yes
Indonesia	no		x		x			x	yes	yes
Maldives	no	x			x	x			no	no
Myanmar	no		x	x		x			no	yes
Nepal	no	x		x				x	yes	no
Sri Lanka	1986[b]	x		x				x	no	yes
Thailand	1989	x		x		x			yes	yes

[a] Compiled from answers by countries to the GPA questionnaire.
[b] STD only.

Table 7
HIV antibody testing[a]

	Laboratory testing facilities at		
	central level	provincial level	district level
Bangladesh	x	x	x
Bhutan	x	x	
India	x	x	
Indonesia	x	x	
Maldives	x		
Myanmar	x	x	
Nepal	x	x	
Sri Lanka	x	x	
Thailand	x	x	x

[a] Compiled from answers by countries to the GPA questionnaire.

The Western Pacific Region

Table 1
Country information

	Total population (thousands)[a]	Population 0-14 years (%)[a]	Population 15-49 years (%)[a]	Population >50 years (%)[a]	Annual growth rate (%)[b]	Urban population (thousands)[b]	Infant mortality rate[b,c]	Life expectancy men[b]	Life expectancy women[b]	Gross national product per capita (US$)[d]	Male literacy rate in 1990[e]	Female literacy rate in 1990[e]
American Samoa	52	–	–	–	–	–	–	–	–	–	–	–
Australia	17 843	22	54	25	1.4	15 182	7	74	80	17 000	–	–
Brunei Darussalam	276	33	52	15	2.2	159	8	72	76	–	–	–
Cambodia	8 997	42	49	9	2.5	1 110	114	50	53	0	–	–
China	1 205 181	27	56	17	1.4	343 762	26	69	73	370	–	–
Cook Islands	17	–	–	–	–	–	–	–	–	–	–	–
Fiji	747	37	51	13	1.0	300	23	70	74	–	–	–
French Polynesia	212	35	53	12	2.3	140	16	68	73	–	–	–
Guam	141	32	54	14	1.7	79	8	73	79	–	–	–
Hong Kong	5 845	20	58	22	0.8	5 531	6	75	80	11 490	–	–
Japan	124 959	17	51	32	0.4	96 992	5	76	82	25 430	–	–
Kiribati	75	–	–	–	–	–	–	–	–	–	–	–
Lao People's Democrat. Rep.	4 605	44	45	10	3.0	939	96	50	53	200	–	–
Malaysia	19 239	38	50	12	2.3	8 735	14	69	73	2 320	87	70
Marshall Islands	51	–	–	–	–	–	–	–	–	–	–	–
Micronesia (Federated States)	459	39	49	11	2.5	229	35	66	70	–	–	–
New Caledonia	175	–	–	–	–	–	–	–	–	–	–	–
New Zealand	3 487	23	53	24	0.9	2 933	8	73	79	12 680	–	–
Niue	2	–	–	–	–	–	–	–	–	–	–	–
Northern Mariana Islands	47	–	–	–	–	–	–	–	–	–	–	–
Palau	–	–	–	–	–	–	–	–	–	–	–	–
Papua New Guinea	4 149	40	50	10	2.3	704	53	55	57	860	65	38
Philippines	66 543	39	50	11	2.1	29 543	39	63	67	730	90	90
Samoa	–	–	–	–	–	–	–	–	–	–	–	–
Singapore	2 798	23	60	18	1.0	2 795	7	72	78	11 160	–	–
Solomon Islands	354	45	46	9	3.3	57	26	69	73	–	–	–
Tokelau	8 926	20	49	32	–0.2	6 206	14	69	75	–	–	–
Tonga	–	–	–	–	–	–	–	–	–	–	–	–
Tuvalu	–	–	–	–	–	–	–	–	–	–	–	–
Vanuatu	–	–	–	–	–	–	–	–	–	–	–	–
Viet Nam	70 902	38	50	13	2.0	14 463	36	62	66	–	92	83

[a] Estimate for 1993. Source: UN Population Division 1992.
[b] WHO estimate for 1993 based on data from UN Population Division 1992.
[c] Per 1000 live births.
[d] Data for 1990. Source: World Bank (STARS) (April 1992).
[e] Source: Statistical Yearbook (UNESCO, 1991).

Table 2
Reporting of HIV and AIDS

	HIV infection first reported[a]	No. of AIDS cases reported		Cumulative no. of AIDS cases reported by 1 July 1993[b]
		1991[b]	1992[b]	
American Samoa	1988	0	0	0
Australia	1985	670	432	3 697
Brunei Darussalam	1986	0	0	2
Cambodia	1991	0	0	0
China	1985	3	3	11
Cook Islands	—	0	0	0
Fiji	1989	1	0	5
French Polynesia	1985	1	3	30
Guam	1985	3	2	14
Hong Kong	1984	15	2	63
Japan	1985	82	90	543
Kiribati	1991	0	0	0
Lao People's Democratic Republic	—	1	0	1
Malaysia	1986	14	40	83
Marshall Islands	—	0	0	2
Micronesia (Federated States of)	1989	0	0	2
New Caledonia	1986	16	4	22
New Zealand	1984	78	50	63
Niue	—	0	0	0
Northern Mariana Islands	1983	0	—	4
Palau	—	0	0	0
Papua New Guinea	1987	13	5	47
Philippines	1985	12	16	92
Samoa	1990	0	0	1
Singapore	1985	12	18	58
Solomon Islands	—	0	0	0
Tokelau	—	0	0	0
Tonga	1987	0	0	4
Tuvalu	—	0	0	0
Vanuatu	—	0	0	0
Viet Nam	1990	0	0	0

[a] Compiled from answers by countries to the GPA questionnaire.
[b] Based on other information reported to WHO/GPA by countries.

Table 3

The National AIDS Committee (NAC) and the National AIDS Programme (NAP)[a]

	National AIDS Committee			
	Year established	Chairman's position	NGOs represented (since)	Full-time NAP manager (since)
American Samoa	1980	Director of Preventive Health	no	1988
Australia	1988	Member of Tribunal for Administrative Appeals	1988	1989
Brunei Darussalam	1988	Minister of Health	no	no
Cambodia	1991	Director, Department of Health	no	no
China	1990	Vice Minister of Public Health	no	1990
Cook Islands	1987	Secretary of Health	1987	no
Fiji	1989	Minister of Health	1989	no
French Polynesia	1986	Director of Public Health	no	no
Guam	1990	—	yes	1988
Hong Kong	1990	Director of Health	1990	1991
Japan	1986	Professor Emiritus, Jantendo University	1986	—
Kiribati	—	Chief of Preventive and Public Health Service, Ministry of Health	yes	—
Lao People's Democratic Rep.	1988	Minister of Public Health	no	no
Malaysia	1985	Director of Health Services	1985	1990
Marshall Islands	1987	Medical Director Preventive Services	1987	no
Micronesia (Federated States of)	1987	Secretary, Department of Human Resources	1990	1988
New Caledonia	1990	Chief of Gynecology, Centre Hospitalier Territoriale (CHT)	1990	1991
New Zealand	1988	Chief Executive, Institute of Social Research and Development	1988	1992
Niue	1992	Director of Health	yes	no
Northern Mariana Islands	1992	—	1992	1991
Palau	1990	Project Coordinator	1990	no
Papua New Guinea	1986	Private physician	1988	1987
Philippines	1987	Undersecretary of Health	no	1987
Samoa	1987	Director General of Health	1987	no
Singapore	1985	Head, Department of Pathology, General Hospital	no	1986
Solomon Islands	1988	Permanent Secretary	1988	no
Tokelau	1990	—	no	no
Tonga	1988	Director of Health	1988	no
Tuvalu	1989	rotating chairmanship	1989	no
Vanuatu	1989	Director of Health	1989	1992
Viet Nam	1990	Minister of Health	1990	no

[a] Compiled from answers by countries to the GPA questionnaire, updated where possible by other information available to GPA in mid-1993.

Table 4

Government departments and ministries implementing AIDS-related activities[a]

	Health	Education & culture	Social welfare & family affairs	Information & media	Interior, home affairs	Women & youth	Armed forces	Finance & planning	Labour	Other
American Samoa	x	x								
Australia	x	x								corrective services
Brunei Darussalam	x			x						Prime Minister's office
Cambodia	x									
China	x									
Cook Islands	x									
Fiji	x	x				x				
French Polynesia	x	x								
Guam	x	x								
Hong Kong	x	x	x	x						narcotics division
Japan	x									government offices
Kiribati	x					x				
Lao People's Democratic Rep.	x									
Malaysia	x	x		x	x					
Marshall Islands	x	x				x				
Micronesia (Federated States of)	x	x				x				
New Caledonia	x	x								
New Zealand	x	—	—	—	—	—	—	—	—	
Niue	x	—	—	—	—	—	—	—	—	
Northern Mariana Islands	x	x				x				Governor's office
Palau	x	x								
Papua New Guinea	x	x			x	x	x			
Philippines	x	x								
Samoa	x					x				
Singapore	x	x			x		x		x	law, national development of trade & industry
Solomon Islands	x									
Tokelau	x									
Tonga	x					x				
Tuvalu	x									
Vanuatu	x	x								
Viet Nam	x	x		x	x	x	x		x	foreign affairs, sport

[a] Compiled from answers by countries to the GPA questionnaire.

Table 5

Supply of condoms

	Condoms distributed (thousands)[a]		Condom social marketing programme in 1992[b]
	1990	1991	
American Samoa	0.6	1.8	no
Australia	15 000[c]	17 000[c]	no
Brunei Darussalam	—	—	no
Cambodia	0	0	no
China	—	—	no
Cook Islands	1	1	no
Fiji	—	—	yes
French Polynesia	—	10	no
Guam	—	—	no
Hong Kong	—	—	no
Japan	—	—	—
Kiribati	2	2	no
Lao People's Democratic Rep.	—	—	no
Malaysia	—	—	no
Marshall Islands	11	12	no
Micronesia (Federated States of)	50	70	no
New Caledonia	—	—	—
New Zealand	—	—	no
Niue	—	—	no
Northern Mariana Islands	—	8	yes
Palau	—	7	no
Papua New Guinea	—	700	yes
Philippines	—	—	yes
Samoa	10	12	yes
Singapore	—	—	yes
Solomon Islands	—	—	yes
Tokelau	0	0	no
Tonga	—	—	yes
Tuvalu	5	10	no
Vanuatu	30	45	yes
Viet Nam	1 500	2 000	yes

[a] Compiled from answers by countries to the GPA questionnaire. The stated number of condoms distributed does not always include those sold by the private sector.

[b] Compiled from answers by countries to the GPA questionnaire and other information available to GPA.

[c] These figures reflect condoms sold.

Table 6
AIDS information, education and communication (IEC)[a]

	AIDS & STD education included in school curricula (since)	Frequency of AIDS messages on:				Free air time given to AIDS messages			Promotion of condoms:	
		radio		television						
		more often than weekly	less often than weekly	more often than weekly	less often than weekly	yes	partly	no	through mass media	to vulnerable groups
American Samoa	1989		x		x		x		yes	yes
Australia	1989		x		x		x		yes	yes
Brunei Darussalam	no		x		x	x			no	yes
Cambodia	no		x		x	x			no	yes
China	1989		x[b]		x[b]		x		no	no
Cook Islands	no	x		x				x	yes	yes
Fiji	—	x						x	no	yes
French Polynesia	1988		x		x	x			yes	yes
Guam	1990	x		x			x		no	no
Hong Kong	1990	x		x		x			yes	yes
Japan	1987	x		x			x		yes	yes
Kiribati	no	—		—		—			—	—
Lao People's Democratic Rep.	no		x				x		no	no
Malaysia	1991	x		x			x		no	yes
Marshall Islands	—	x		x		x			yes	yes
Micronesia (Federated States of)	1991	x		x		x			yes	yes
New Caledonia	1991		x	x				x	yes	yes
New Zealand	1990		x		x			x	no	yes
Niue	no		x		x			x	no	no
Northern Mariana Islands	1992	x		x		x			yes	yes
Palau	1991		x		x	x			yes	yes
Papua New Guinea	1989		x		x		x		no	yes
Philippines	no		x		x			x	yes	yes
Samoa	1991	x						x	no	yes
Singapore	1986		x[c]		x[c]			x	yes	yes
Solomon Islands	no		x					x	yes	yes
Tokelau	no	—		—				x	no	yes
Tonga	1989	x						x	—	yes
Tuvalu	no	x				x			no	yes
Vanuatu	no	x				x			yes	yes
Viet Nam	1991		x		x	x			yes	yes

[a] Compiled from answers by countries to a GPA questionnaire.
[b] Around World AIDS Day.
[c] Publicity blitz in November and December.

Table 7
HIV antibody testing[a]

	Laboratory testing facilities at		
	central level	provincial level	district level
American Samoa	x		
Australia	x	x	x
Brunei Darussalam	x	x	
Cambodia	x		
China	x	x	
Cook Islands	x	x	
Fiji	x	x	x
French Polynesia	x	x	x
Guam	x		
Hong Kong	x		
Japan	x	x	x
Kiribati	x		
Lao People's Democratic Rep.	x	x	
Malaysia	x	x	x
Marshall Islands	x		
Micronesia (Federated States of)	x	x	
New Caledonia	x		
New Zealand	x	x	
Niue	x		
Northern Mariana Islands	x		
Palau	x		
Papua New Guinea	x	x	
Philippines	x	x	
Samoa	x	x	
Singapore	x	x	
Solomon Islands	x		
Tokelau		—	
Tonga	x	x	
Tuvalu	x		
Vanuatu	x	x	x
Viet Nam	x	x	

[a] Compiled from answers by countries to the GPA questionnaire.